Group Therapy Activities for Psychiatric Nursing

A Complete, Practical, Evidence-Based Guide to Leading Therapeutic Groups

Mabel Stephanie Hale and Keeran Launcelot Mitchell

Copyright © 2025 by Mabel Stephanie Hale and Keeran Launcelot Mitchell

All rights reserved. No part of this publication may be reproduced, distributed, or transmitted in any form or by any means, including photocopying, recording, or other electronic or mechanical methods, without the prior written permission of the copyright holders, except in the case of brief quotations embodied in critical reviews and certain other noncommercial uses permitted by copyright law.

Clinical Worksheets and Assessment Tools Usage: The worksheets, assessment forms, and clinical templates contained in this book are provided for use by qualified healthcare professionals with their patients in clinical practice. Healthcare providers may reproduce these materials for direct patient care purposes only. Any other reproduction, distribution, or commercial use requires written permission from the copyright holders.

Educational Use: Limited reproduction of excerpts is permitted for educational purposes in accredited healthcare training programs, provided proper attribution is given and use is non-commercial.

First Edition: 2025

ISBN: 978-1-7641941-9-8

Isohan Publishing

The information contained in this book is intended for qualified healthcare professionals and is provided for educational purposes only. The authors and publisher disclaim any liability arising directly or indirectly from the use of this book.

The interventions and activities described in this book should only be implemented by licensed mental health professionals within their scope of practice. Readers are responsible for ensuring compliance with local regulations, institutional policies, and professional licensing requirements.

Clinical Responsibility Disclaimer

All clinical interventions must be adapted to individual patient needs and circumstances. The authors and publisher assume no responsibility for patient outcomes resulting from use of materials contained in this book. Healthcare providers must exercise their professional judgment and clinical expertise when implementing any interventions described.

Names And Case Examples Disclaimer

All patient names, case examples, and clinical scenarios presented in this book are fictional composites created for educational purposes. Any resemblance to actual persons, living or deceased, or actual clinical situations is purely coincidental. No real patient information or confidential healthcare data has been used in the creation of this content.

Table of Contents

Chapter 1: Introduction to Group Therapy in Psychiatric Nursing 1
    Historical Evolution of Group Work in Psychiatric Settings 1
    The Evidence Foundation for Group Interventions 2
    Scope of Practice and Professional Standards 2
    Case Example: Sarah's Journey Through Depression Group 3
    Case Example: Managing Crisis in Anxiety Group 4
    Case Example: Trauma Processing in Mixed Diagnostic Group 4
    Integration with Interdisciplinary Treatment Teams 5
    Measuring Group Therapy Effectiveness 6
    Practical Considerations for New Group Facilitators 7
    Ethical Considerations in Group Practice 7
    Key Learning Points 8

Chapter 2: Nursing Theoretical Frameworks for Group Practice 9
    Peplau's Interpersonal Relations Theory in Group Context 9
    Orlando's Deliberative Nursing Process Applied to Groups 10
    Case Example: Applying Peplau's Theory with Adolescent Group 11
    Case Example: Orlando's Deliberative Process During Group Crisis 12
    Case Example: Integrating Multiple Nursing Theories 13
    Travelbee's Human-to-Human Relationship Model 14
    Watson's Caring Theory in Group Practice 15
    Practical Integration Strategies 15
    Addressing Complex Group Dynamics 16
    Moving Forward with Confidence 16
    Essential Takeaways 17

Chapter 3: Group Dynamics and Therapeutic Factors 18

    Yalom's Therapeutic Factors in Nursing Practice 18

    Group Development Stages and Nursing Interventions 20

    Case Example: Managing Resistance in Early Recovery Group.................................21

    Case Example: Facilitating Therapeutic Factors in Trauma Group 22

    Case Example: Crisis Management During Group Conflict.......................................24

    Creating Psychological Safety 24

    Managing Challenging Dynamics 25

    Measuring Group Effectiveness 26

    Building Your Skills 26

    Core Insights for Practice 27

Chapter 4: Cognitive Behavioral Therapy (CBT) Groups for Nurses 28

    Core CBT Principles for Group Application..28

    Thought Records Adapted for Groups 29

    Case Example: Thought Record Group for Depression 30

    Cognitive Restructuring Exercises..31

    Behavioral Activation Planning 32

    Case Example: Behavioral Activation for Anxiety Group 32

    Case Example: Problem-Solving Skills Training 33

    Nursing-Specific CBT Adaptations 35

    Documentation Templates and Progress Tracking 35

    Building CBT Group Facilitation Skills 36

    Preparing for Advanced Applications 37

    Practice-Ready Skills..38

Chapter 5: Dialectical Behavior Therapy (DBT) Skills Groups 39

    Understanding the DBT Framework...39

    Mindfulness Skills Module...40

    Case Example: Mindfulness Skills with Trauma Survivors.......................................41

    Distress Tolerance Skills Module 42

- Emotion Regulation Skills Module 43
- Case Example: Emotion Regulation with Bipolar Disorder 43
- Interpersonal Effectiveness Skills Module 45
- Case Example: Interpersonal Skills with Social Anxiety 45
- Nursing Adaptations for Inpatient Settings 47
- Outcome Measurement and Progress Tracking 47
- Building Toward Advanced Practice 48
- Sustainable Practice 49
- Foundational Insights 49

Chapter 6: Mindfulness and Stress Reduction Groups 50
- Evidence Base for Mindfulness in Psychiatric Nursing 50
- Progressive Muscle Relaxation Scripts 51
- Case Example: Progressive Muscle Relaxation for Chronic Pain Group 51
- Guided Imagery Exercises 53
- Breathing Techniques for Anxiety 53
- Case Example: Breathing Techniques for Panic Disorder 54
- Case Example: Walking Meditation for Depression Group 55
- Safety Considerations for Dissociative Disorders 56
- Integration with Medication Management 57
- Building Sustainable Practice 58
- Wisdom for Practice 58
- Essential Learning Elements 59

Chapter 7: Psychopharmacology Education Groups 60
- Patient Medication Education Groups Framework 60
- Understanding Psychiatric Medications Module 61
- Case Example: Antidepressant Education for First-Episode Depression 62
- Side Effect Management Strategies Module 63
- Drug Interactions and Safety Module 64

Case Example: Mood Stabilizer Education for Bipolar Disorder 64
Case Example: Antipsychotic Education for Schizophrenia 66
Long-Acting Injectable Education Module 67
Interactive Teaching Methods 67
Health Literacy Adaptations 68
Building Collaborative Relationships 69
Looking Beyond the Group 69
Practical Wisdom 70
Core Learning Elements 70

Chapter 8: Medication Adherence and Compliance Groups 71
Evidence-Based Adherence Interventions 71
Medication Calendars and Tracking Sheets 72
Case Example: Adherence Support for Bipolar Disorder 72
Problem-Solving Adherence Barriers 74
Peer Support Strategies 74
Case Example: Peer Support for Depression Treatment 75
Case Example: Technology Integration for Schizophrenia 76
Cultural Considerations in Medication Beliefs 77
Family Involvement Strategies 78
Technology Integration Solutions 79
Measuring Adherence Outcomes 79
Sustaining Motivation 80
Key Implementation Strategies 81

Chapter 9: Adolescent Psychiatric Group Interventions 82
Integrated Model Combining Interpersonal and Feminist Perspectives 82
Creative Arts Therapy Adaptations 83
Case Example: Creative Arts for Adolescent Depression Group 84
Social Skills Training Adaptations 85

    Technology-Assisted Interventions 86

    Case Example: Technology Integration for Social Anxiety 86

    Case Example: Peer Support Groups for Eating Disorders 87

    School Liaison and Transition Planning 88

    Safety Protocols for Self-Harm Behaviors 89

    Family Involvement Strategies 90

    Developmental Considerations 91

    Building Resilience 91

    Pathways to Success 92

    Clinical Applications 92

Chapter 10: Geriatric Mental Health Groups 94

    Evidence Base for Geriatric Group Therapy 94

    Reminiscence Therapy Protocols 95

    Case Example: Reminiscence Therapy for Late-Life Depression 95

    Cognitive Stimulation Activities 97

    Grief and Loss Support Groups 97

    Case Example: Grief Support Following Spouse Loss 98

    Case Example: Anxiety Management in Late Life 99

    Social Engagement Programs 100

    Environmental Modifications 101

    Collaboration with Long-Term Care 101

    Medical Integration 102

    Cultural Considerations for Older Adults 103

    Wisdom Through Experience 103

    Essential Implementation Elements 104

Chapter 11: Dual Diagnosis Group Interventions 105

    Integrated Treatment Approaches 105

    Triggers and Coping Skills Worksheets 106

  Case Example: Integrated Treatment for Depression and Alcohol Use Disorder 106
  Relapse Prevention Planning 108
  Recovery Support Groups 108
  Case Example: Relapse Prevention for Bipolar Disorder and Cocaine Use 109
  Case Example: Trauma-Informed Approach for PTSD and Alcohol Use 110
  Motivational Interviewing Techniques 111
  Medication-Assisted Treatment Education 111
  Trauma-Informed Approaches 112
  Family and Social System Interventions 113
  Building Integrated Recovery 113
  Clinical Integration Points 114

Chapter 12: Cultural Competency in Group Practice 115
  Cultural Competency Framework 115
  Cultural Assessment Tools 116
  Case Example: Culturally Adapted Depression Group for Latina Women 116
  Language and Communication Adaptations 117
  Incorporating Cultural Healers 118
  Case Example: Integration of Traditional Healing for Native American Veterans 119
  Case Example: Islamic Cultural Adaptations for Anxiety Treatment 120
  Religious and Spiritual Considerations 121
  Interpreter Use in Groups 121
  LGBTQIA+ Cultural Competency 122
  Socioeconomic Cultural Factors 123
  Building Cultural Bridges 123
  Reflections on Diversity 124
  Cultural Practice Foundations 124

Chapter 13: Group Facilitation Skills for Nurses 126
- Leadership Styles in Group Therapy 126
- Opening and Closing Rituals 127
- Case Example: Opening Rituals for Trauma Recovery Group 128
- Managing Dominant Members 128
- Encouraging Quiet Participants 129
- Case Example: Balancing Participation in Depression Group 130
- Case Example: Managing Emotional Intensity in Anxiety Group 131
- Handling Emotional Intensity 132
- Co-Facilitation Models 132
- Supervision and Consultation 133
- Time Management Strategies 134
- Building Therapeutic Relationships 134
- Technology Integration 135
- Practical Applications 136
- Foundational Skills 136

Chapter 14: Safety and Crisis Management in Groups 137
- Environmental Safety Protocols 137
- Risk Assessment Procedures 138
- Case Example: Managing Suicidal Crisis in Depression Group 138
- De-escalation Scripts 139
- Safety Planning Worksheets 140
- Case Example: De-escalation for Bipolar Group Crisis 141
- Case Example: Medical Emergency Response 141
- Emergency Response Protocols 142
- Post-Crisis Debriefing 143
- Legal and Ethical Considerations 144
- Incident Documentation 144

    Training and Competency Development 145

    Building Crisis Resilience 146

    Practice Wisdom 146

    Emergency Management Essentials 147

Chapter 15: Program Development and Evaluation 148

    Needs Assessment Strategies 148

    Logic Models for Groups 149

    Case Example: Developing Adolescent Depression Program 149

    Budget Planning Worksheets 150

    Staffing Calculations 151

    Case Example: Implementing Dual Diagnosis Program 152

    Case Example: Geriatric Mental Health Program Development 153

    Space and Resource Requirements 154

    Continuous Quality Improvement 154

    Sustainability Planning 155

    Marketing and Outreach 156

    Program Evaluation Methods 156

    Innovation and Adaptation 157

    Program Building Blocks 158

Chapter 16: Psychoeducational Groups for Specific Disorders 159

    Depression Education Groups 159

    Case Example: Depression Education for Postpartum Group 160

    Anxiety and Panic Disorder Groups 161

    Case Example: Panic Disorder Education for Workplace Group 161

    Bipolar Disorder Management Groups 162

    Case Example: Bipolar Education for College Students 163

    Schizophrenia and Psychosis Education Groups 164

    PTSD and Trauma Groups 164

Case Example: PTSD Education for Veterans Group 165
Personality Disorder Skills Training 166
Adapting Teaching Methods for Symptoms 166
Case Example: Adapting Education for Cognitive Impairment 167
Measuring Knowledge Acquisition 168
Cultural Adaptations for Education 168
Technology Integration 169
Building Treatment Motivation 169
Moving Forward with Knowledge 170
Educational Foundations 170

Chapter 17: Integrating Groups with Nursing Care Plans 172

Care Plan Integration Strategies 172
Case Example: Integrating Depression Group with Individual Care Plans 173
Documentation Systems 174
Case Example: Documentation for Dual Diagnosis Integration 174
Interdisciplinary Communication 175
Case Example: Interdisciplinary Integration for Trauma Recovery 176
Outcome Tracking Across Settings 177
Technology Support for Integration 177
Addressing Integration Challenges 178
Quality Improvement Initiatives 179
Training and Development 179
Sustainability and Growth 180
Integration Essentials 181

Chapter 18: Ready-to-Use Worksheets and Clinical Tools 182

CBT Thought Records and Activity Logs 182
Worksheet CBT-1: Basic Thought Record 182
Worksheet CBT-2: Daily Activity Log 183

Worksheet CBT-3: Behavioral Experiment Planning ... 183
Worksheet CBT-4: Problem-Solving Worksheet ... 184
Worksheet CBT-5: Mood and Thought Monitoring ... 185
DBT Skills Practice Sheets ... 186
Worksheet DBT-1: Mindfulness Skills Practice Log ... 186
Worksheet DBT-2: Distress Tolerance Skills Tracker ... 186
Worksheet DBT-3: Emotion Regulation Worksheet ... 187
Worksheet DBT-4: Interpersonal Effectiveness Planning ... 188
Worksheet DBT-5: Daily Skills Review ... 189
Mindfulness Exercise Scripts ... 190
Worksheet MIN-1: Progressive Muscle Relaxation Script ... 190
Worksheet MIN-2: Body Scan Meditation Guide ... 191
Worksheet MIN-3: Breathing Exercise Instructions ... 191
Worksheet MIN-4: Mindful Walking Instructions ... 192
Worksheet MIN-5: Five Senses Grounding Exercise ... 193
Medication Tracking Forms ... 195
Worksheet MED-1: Daily Medication and Mood Log ... 195
Worksheet MED-2: Weekly Medication Review ... 195
Worksheet MED-3: Side Effect Monitoring Form ... 196
Worksheet MED-4: Medication Change Tracking ... 197
Worksheet MED-5: Medication Adherence Problem-Solving ... 198
Safety Planning Templates ... 199
Worksheet SAFE-1: Personal Safety Plan ... 199
Worksheet SAFE-2: Crisis Contact Card ... 200
Worksheet SAFE-3: Self-Harm Alternative Strategies ... 201
Worksheet SAFE-4: Emergency Action Plan ... 202
Worksheet SAFE-5: Recovery Wellness Plan ... 202
Cultural Assessment Tools ... 204

Worksheet CULT-1: Cultural Background Assessment 204
Worksheet CULT-2: Religious and Spiritual Assessment 205
Worksheet CULT-3: Family Cultural Dynamics 206
Worksheet CULT-4: Acculturation Assessment 207
Worksheet CULT-5: Preferred Cultural Interventions 208
Group Evaluation Forms 210
Worksheet EVAL-1: Session Feedback Form 210
Worksheet EVAL-2: Group Climate Assessment 211
Worksheet EVAL-3: Therapeutic Factors Inventory 212
Worksheet EVAL-4: Individual Progress Review 213
Worksheet EVAL-5: Program Completion Survey 214
Implementation Guidelines 216
Essential Worksheet Applications 216

Appendix A: Reproducible Worksheets and Handouts 217
CBT Thought Records and Activity Logs 217
Case Example: Thought Record Implementation in Anxiety Group 218
DBT Skills Practice Sheets 219
Mindfulness Exercise Scripts 219
Case Example: Mindfulness Scripts for PTSD Group 220
Medication Tracking Forms 221
Safety Planning Templates 221
Case Example: Safety Planning for Borderline Personality Group 222
Cultural Assessment Tools 223
Group Evaluation Forms 224
Creating Effective Worksheets 224
Distribution and Follow-up 225
Resource Development 225
Essential Resource Components 226

Appendix B: Assessment Tools and Outcome Measures 227
Beck Depression Inventory (BDI-II) 227
GAD-7 Anxiety Scale 228
Patient Health Questionnaire (PHQ-9) 228
Case Example: Integrating Multiple Assessment Tools 229
Health of the Nation Outcome Scales (HoNOS) 230
Group Cohesion Scales 231
Session Rating Scales 231
Treatment Satisfaction Surveys 232
Case Example: Comprehensive Outcome Measurement 232
Selecting Appropriate Measures 233
Data Management and Analysis 234
Building Assessment Culture 234
Measurement Foundations 235

Appendix C: Documentation Templates 236
Group Progress Note Formats 236
Case Example: SOAP Documentation Implementation 237
Attendance Tracking Sheets 237
Behavioral Observation Forms 238
Incident Report Templates 239
Case Example: Incident Documentation for Group Crisis 239
Outcome Summary Reports 240
Insurance Documentation Guides 240
Case Example: Insurance Documentation Strategy 241
Electronic Documentation Systems 242
Legal and Ethical Considerations 242
Documentation Training and Support 243
Moving Forward with Documentation 243

Documentation Essentials 244
Reference **245**

Chapter 1: Introduction to Group Therapy in Psychiatric Nursing

The practice of group therapy in psychiatric nursing represents one of the most powerful yet underutilized tools in contemporary mental health care. While individual therapy sessions often receive the spotlight, the unique dynamics and therapeutic potential of group interventions offer psychiatric nurses extraordinary opportunities to create lasting change in their patients' lives. You stand at the intersection of nursing science and group psychology, equipped with both clinical expertise and the interpersonal skills necessary to guide multiple individuals toward healing simultaneously.

Historical Evolution of Group Work in Psychiatric Settings

The roots of group therapy in psychiatric nursing stretch back to the early 20th century, though the formalization of these practices took decades to develop. Initially, group activities in psychiatric hospitals served primarily custodial purposes—keeping patients occupied rather than providing therapeutic benefit. However, pioneering nurses recognized the potential for structured group interactions to promote recovery and social reintegration.

During World War II, the shortage of individual therapists led to innovative group approaches that demonstrated remarkable effectiveness. Psychiatric nurses found themselves naturally positioned to lead these groups, given their round-the-clock presence with patients and their understanding of both medical and psychosocial needs. This historical moment marked the beginning of formal recognition for nurses as group therapy facilitators.

The development accelerated through the 1960s and 1970s as deinstitutionalization created new demands for community-based group interventions. Nurses working in outpatient settings, partial hospitalization programs, and community mental health centers began developing structured group protocols that addressed specific psychiatric conditions and populations.

Today, psychiatric nurses lead groups in diverse settings—from acute inpatient units to intensive outpatient programs, from school-based mental health services to geriatric care facilities. This evolution reflects not just historical circumstance but the unique qualifications nurses bring to group facilitation: clinical knowledge, 24-hour patient perspective, and the nursing profession's holistic approach to care.

The Evidence Foundation for Group Interventions

Research consistently demonstrates that group therapy can be as effective as individual therapy for many psychiatric conditions, and in some cases, superior. A comprehensive meta-analysis of 329 randomized controlled trials revealed effect sizes for group interventions ranging from 0.58 to 0.89, indicating moderate to large therapeutic benefits across diverse populations and conditions (1).

These findings hold particular significance for psychiatric nurses because they validate what many have observed clinically: patients often make breakthroughs in group settings that prove elusive in individual sessions. The research shows specific advantages for group approaches, including enhanced social learning, peer support, reduced isolation, and cost-effectiveness that makes treatment accessible to more individuals.

For anxiety disorders, group cognitive-behavioral therapy shows effect sizes comparable to individual treatment while providing the added benefit of exposure to social situations that trigger anxiety. Depression treatment groups demonstrate sustained improvements that often exceed individual therapy outcomes, particularly regarding social functioning and relationship skills.

Perhaps most striking, substance use disorder treatment shows consistently better outcomes when delivered in group formats. The peer support, accountability, and shared experience inherent in group settings address core aspects of addiction that individual therapy cannot replicate.

Scope of Practice and Professional Standards

Psychiatric nurses practicing group therapy operate within clearly defined professional boundaries while exercising considerable autonomy in group design and implementation. The American Psychiatric Nurses Association recognizes group therapy as within the scope of practice for registered nurses with appropriate training and experience.

Your role as a group facilitator differs significantly from that of other mental health professionals. While psychologists and social workers often focus primarily on psychological interventions, you bring medical knowledge, medication expertise, and holistic nursing assessment to group work. This unique perspective allows you to identify medical issues affecting group participation, educate about medication effects, and integrate physical health considerations into group interventions.

Professional standards require that you maintain competency through continuing education, seek supervision when appropriate, and practice within your scope of knowledge and experience. Most healthcare systems require specific training in group therapy techniques before nurses can independently facilitate therapeutic groups.

Documentation requirements for group therapy mirror those for individual interventions but include additional considerations such as group dynamics, individual responses within the group context, and progress toward both individual and group goals. You must balance confidentiality requirements with the shared nature of group participation, ensuring that progress notes protect individual privacy while capturing the therapeutic value of group interactions.

Case Example: Sarah's Journey Through Depression Group

Sarah, a 34-year-old accountant, entered our 12-week depression treatment group following her third hospitalization for major depressive disorder. Despite multiple trials of antidepressant medications and individual therapy, she continued to struggle with persistent hopelessness and social withdrawal.

During the initial group session, Sarah sat silently in the corner, making minimal eye contact and contributing only when directly addressed. Her body language communicated defeat—slumped shoulders, downcast eyes, and defensive arm positioning. As the group facilitator, I recognized these patterns as common initial presentations but also noted Sarah's keen attention to other members' stories.

By week four, Sarah began sharing her experiences with medication side effects, which resonated strongly with other group members. This seemingly simple contribution marked a turning point—she had found a way to help others while beginning to voice her own struggles. The group's response was overwhelmingly supportive, with several members sharing similar experiences and coping strategies.

The transformation accelerated through weeks six through ten. Sarah began arriving early to chat with other members, volunteered to help with group activities, and started using humor to cope with difficult emotions. Most significantly, she began challenging other members' negative thinking patterns, a process that helped her recognize and modify her own cognitive distortions.

By group completion, Sarah demonstrated marked improvement not just in depression scores but in social functioning and self-efficacy. She had developed genuine friendships with three group members and was exploring volunteer opportunities in her community. The group experience provided something individual therapy had not—proof that she could connect with others, contribute meaningfully to relationships, and find purpose beyond her own recovery.

Case Example: Managing Crisis in Anxiety Group

During a routine anxiety management group session, Michael, a 28-year-old graduate student, experienced a severe panic attack triggered by a discussion about upcoming exams. His symptoms included hyperventilation, chest pain, trembling, and expressions of fear about dying or losing control.

The group's initial reaction was mixed—some members became anxious themselves, others wanted to help but didn't know how, and a few seemed to withdraw from the situation. As the nurse facilitator, I needed to manage both Michael's immediate crisis and the group's response to maintain therapeutic safety for all members.

First, I implemented immediate interventions for Michael—guided breathing exercises, grounding techniques, and reassurance about the temporary nature of panic symptoms. Simultaneously, I addressed the group by explaining what was happening and normalizing their various reactions to witnessing someone else's distress.

The crisis became a powerful learning opportunity. Group members who had previously minimized their own anxiety symptoms gained new understanding of anxiety's physical manifestations. Several members shared their own panic experiences, creating unexpected bonds and reducing stigma around anxiety symptoms.

Michael's response to the group's support during his vulnerable moment became a catalyst for his recovery. He had expected rejection or judgment but instead found acceptance and understanding. This experience challenged his core belief that others would abandon him if they saw his anxiety, leading to significant improvement in his social anxiety and willingness to seek support.

The incident also strengthened overall group cohesion. Members developed a shared understanding of anxiety's impact and greater confidence in their ability to support each other through difficult moments. The group established new norms around crisis support and developed protocols for managing anxiety symptoms together.

Case Example: Trauma Processing in Mixed Diagnostic Group

Elena, a 45-year-old teacher with PTSD following a car accident, joined our mixed diagnostic group that included members with depression, anxiety, and bipolar disorder. Initially, there was concern about including someone with trauma symptoms in a general group, but Elena specifically requested this setting over trauma-specific groups.

During week three, Elena shared details about intrusive memories and nightmares related to her accident. Her disclosure prompted unexpected responses from other group members—several revealed their own trauma histories, including childhood abuse, domestic violence, and military service. What emerged was recognition that trauma underlies many psychiatric conditions, even when not explicitly identified as the primary diagnosis.

The group naturally developed trauma-informed approaches to their interactions. Members became sensitive to triggers, learned grounding techniques together, and created agreements about supporting each other during flashbacks or dissociative episodes. Elena's openness about trauma normalized these experiences for others and reduced shame around trauma symptoms.

Elena's progress accelerated through group participation in ways that individual therapy had not achieved. The group provided multiple perspectives on recovery, various coping strategies, and evidence that healing was possible. She observed other members managing their symptoms successfully, which increased her hope and motivation for recovery.

By group completion, Elena had returned to work, resumed driving, and developed a robust support network. More importantly, she had processed her trauma within a context of connection rather than isolation, demonstrating the power of group interventions to address complex psychiatric presentations.

Integration with Interdisciplinary Treatment Teams

Group therapy in psychiatric settings rarely occurs in isolation but rather as part of coordinated treatment planning involving multiple disciplines. Your role as nurse-group facilitator positions you uniquely to bridge different aspects of patient care and communicate group insights to the broader treatment team.

Regular communication with psychiatrists ensures that group observations inform medication decisions. Patients often display different behaviors in group settings compared to individual appointments, providing valuable information about social functioning, medication effects, and symptom patterns. You might observe medication side effects that become apparent only during group activities or notice therapeutic responses that patients don't report in individual sessions.

Collaboration with social workers focuses on discharge planning and community resource connections. Group therapy often reveals practical needs and social deficits that require targeted interventions. You can identify patients who would benefit from specific community groups, family therapy, or social services while also preparing them for transitions from inpatient to outpatient care.

Coordination with occupational therapists, recreational therapists, and other rehabilitation professionals ensures that group therapy goals align with overall treatment objectives. Your observations about patients' functional abilities, social skills, and cognitive functioning in group settings inform treatment planning across disciplines.

Case managers rely on your group assessments to understand patients' readiness for discharge, community placement decisions, and ongoing service needs. Group participation often provides the most accurate assessment of patients' social functioning and ability to engage in community-based services.

Measuring Group Therapy Effectiveness

Evaluation of group therapy outcomes requires both individual and group-level measurements. You must track each member's progress toward personal treatment goals while also monitoring group dynamics, cohesion, and collective therapeutic factors.

Individual outcome measures include standardized assessment tools administered before, during, and after group participation. Common instruments include the Beck Depression Inventory, Generalized Anxiety Disorder scale, and functional assessment measures that capture changes in daily living skills and social functioning.

Group-level measures focus on therapeutic factors, group cohesion, and collective progress indicators. The Group Climate Questionnaire assesses member perceptions of group engagement, avoidance, and conflict. Cohesion measures evaluate the strength of bonds between members and their commitment to group goals.

Process measures examine attendance patterns, participation levels, and specific therapeutic events that occur during group sessions. You document critical incidents, breakthrough moments, and patterns of interaction that contribute to or hinder therapeutic progress.

Long-term follow-up data provides the most meaningful evaluation of group therapy effectiveness. Many benefits of group participation—improved social skills, enhanced support networks, and increased help-seeking behaviors—become apparent only months after group completion.

Practical Considerations for New Group Facilitators

Beginning group therapy practice requires careful attention to practical details that support therapeutic success. Room setup affects group dynamics significantly—circular seating arrangements promote equality and eye contact, while the presence of clocks, tissues, and comfort items demonstrates preparation and care.

Group size optimization balances multiple factors including therapeutic goals, member characteristics, and facilitator experience. Smaller groups (4-6 members) allow for deeper exploration of individual issues, while larger groups (8-12 members) provide more diverse perspectives and social learning opportunities.

Timing considerations include session length, frequency, and duration of group treatment. Most therapy groups meet weekly for 60-90 minutes over 8-16 weeks, though acute inpatient groups may meet daily for shorter durations. Consistency in scheduling builds routine and predictability that supports therapeutic engagement.

Screening procedures ensure appropriate group composition and member readiness for group participation. You evaluate potential members' cognitive abilities, social functioning, and specific contraindications such as active psychosis, severe personality disorders, or crisis states that require individual attention.

Ethical Considerations in Group Practice

Group therapy presents unique ethical challenges that require careful navigation. Confidentiality becomes complex when multiple individuals share personal information in group settings. You must establish clear guidelines about what information can be shared outside the group while recognizing that you cannot guarantee other members will maintain confidentiality.

Dual relationships become particularly problematic in group settings where members may develop personal relationships that extend beyond the therapeutic context. Clear boundaries must be established regarding contact between group members outside of sessions and your role in managing these relationships.

Informed consent for group therapy includes additional considerations such as the presence of other group members, the possibility of encountering other members in community settings, and the different therapeutic approach compared to individual treatment.

Crisis management in groups requires protocols for managing suicidal ideation, violence risk, or psychiatric emergencies when other group members are present. You must balance individual safety needs with group therapeutic goals and the psychological impact on other members.

Group therapy represents both an art and a science—requiring technical knowledge of therapeutic techniques combined with intuitive understanding of human relationships and group dynamics. Your success as a group facilitator depends on continuous learning, regular supervision, and willingness to adapt your approach based on group needs and emerging research.

The chapters that follow will provide specific frameworks, techniques, and interventions that transform group therapy knowledge into effective clinical practice. Each theoretical model and practical skill builds upon this foundation of understanding about the unique role psychiatric nurses play in group therapeutic settings.

Your patients need what group therapy offers—connection, hope, shared learning, and evidence that recovery is possible. You have the clinical knowledge, interpersonal skills, and professional commitment necessary to facilitate these powerful therapeutic experiences.

Key Learning Points

- Psychiatric nurses bring unique qualifications to group therapy including medical knowledge, holistic assessment skills, and 24-hour patient perspective
- Research demonstrates group therapy effectiveness equal to or superior than individual treatment for many psychiatric conditions
- Professional practice requires specific training, appropriate supervision, and adherence to scope of practice guidelines
- Group crisis management requires simultaneous attention to individual safety and group therapeutic needs
- Integration with interdisciplinary teams enhances both group therapy outcomes and overall treatment planning
- Ethical considerations in group practice include complex confidentiality issues, boundary management, and informed consent procedures

Chapter 2: Nursing Theoretical Frameworks for Group Practice

Theoretical frameworks provide the foundation for effective group therapy practice, transforming random collection of interventions into purposeful, evidence-based treatment approaches. Nursing theories offer unique perspectives on group work that distinguish your practice from other mental health professionals—perspectives that emphasize relationship, holistic care, and the inherent capacity for healing that exists within every individual.

You don't simply apply psychological theories to group settings; instead, you draw upon nursing's rich theoretical heritage to create group experiences that reflect nursing's core values and clinical expertise. These frameworks guide your understanding of how therapeutic relationships develop in group contexts, how to address both individual and collective needs, and how to facilitate healing processes that extend beyond symptom reduction to encompass whole-person wellness.

Peplau's Interpersonal Relations Theory in Group Context

Hildegard Peplau's groundbreaking work on interpersonal relationships provides a robust framework for understanding and facilitating group therapy processes. Her theory's emphasis on the nurse-patient relationship as the cornerstone of therapeutic intervention translates powerfully to group settings, where multiple therapeutic relationships develop simultaneously.

The four phases of Peplau's theory—orientation, identification, exploitation, and resolution—manifest differently in group contexts compared to individual relationships, requiring adaptation of interventions while maintaining the theory's core principles (2). Understanding these phases helps you recognize where individual group members are in their therapeutic journeys and how to support both individual progress and group development.

During the **orientation phase**, group members experience anxiety about joining an unknown situation with unfamiliar people. Your role involves reducing this anxiety through clear communication about group expectations, modeling of therapeutic communication, and creation of psychological safety. Unlike individual therapy orientation, group orientation requires attention to member-to-member relationships as well as member-to-facilitator connections.

You facilitate introductions that help members begin to see commonalities while respecting individual uniqueness. This phase often includes establishing group rules, explaining confidentiality expectations, and addressing initial concerns about group participation. The orientation may take several sessions as members adjust to the group format and begin to trust both you and each other.

The **identification phase** in group therapy involves members beginning to recognize similarities with others while developing their unique identity within the group. Members start to see how their experiences relate to others' stories, leading to decreased isolation and increased hope. Your role shifts from primarily educational to more facilitative as members begin to support each other.

During identification, you help members recognize their strengths and resources while acknowledging their struggles. The group setting provides multiple opportunities for identification—members may identify with different aspects of various group members' experiences rather than identifying primarily with you as the facilitator.

The **exploitation phase** represents the working stage of group therapy, when members actively use group resources to address their problems and achieve their goals. Members take more responsibility for group content and support each other's growth. Your role becomes less directive as members develop skills in providing feedback, emotional support, and practical suggestions to each other.

This phase demonstrates the unique power of group interventions—members learn not just from your expertise but from each other's experiences, perspectives, and coping strategies. The exploitation phase often produces the most significant therapeutic breakthroughs as members apply new insights and skills both within the group and in their daily lives.

The **resolution phase** involves preparing for group termination and consolidating gains made during group participation. Members review their progress, identify skills they've developed, and plan for maintaining changes after group completion. Your role includes facilitating closure processes, addressing termination anxiety, and helping members plan for ongoing support.

Orlando's Deliberative Nursing Process Applied to Groups

Ida Orlando's theory of the deliberative nursing process offers a framework for moment-to-moment group facilitation that emphasizes validation, mutual understanding, and immediate response to therapeutic needs (3). Her focus on the nursing process—perception, thought, and feeling leading to action—provides guidance for managing complex group dynamics and responding to multiple needs simultaneously.

Orlando's emphasis on **validation** becomes particularly important in group settings where multiple perspectives and experiences converge. You continuously validate members' experiences while helping them understand how their perceptions may differ from others' viewpoints. This validation process builds trust and encourages authentic participation.

The **deliberative process** involves carefully observing group member behaviors, thoughts, and feelings, then responding in ways that promote therapeutic progress. In group settings, you must track multiple individuals' responses while managing overall group dynamics—a complex skill that develops through practice and supervision.

Orlando's focus on **immediate needs** translates to responsive group facilitation that addresses emerging issues as they arise rather than rigidly following predetermined agendas. When a group member becomes distressed, faces a crisis, or experiences a breakthrough, you adjust group focus to address these immediate therapeutic opportunities.

Case Example: Applying Peplau's Theory with Adolescent Group

The adolescent depression group at our outpatient clinic demonstrated classic Peplau phases over their 16-week treatment period. During orientation, the six teenagers (ages 14-17) showed typical adolescent resistance—eye rolling, minimal verbal participation, and obvious skepticism about group therapy's potential benefits.

Jake, a 16-year-old with major depression following his parents' divorce, exemplified orientation phase challenges. He attended sessions reluctantly, spoke only when directly addressed, and frequently checked his phone despite group rules. His body language communicated clear messages: "I don't want to be here, and I don't think this will help."

My initial interventions focused on reducing Jake's anxiety about group participation rather than confronting his resistance directly. I acknowledged that group therapy felt uncomfortable for most teenagers and validated his uncertainty about sharing personal information with peers. Gradually, Jake began making minimal contributions—answering direct questions and occasionally making humorous comments that showed he was listening to other members.

The identification phase emerged around week five when Sarah, a 15-year-old with depression and anxiety, shared her struggles with her parents' expectations about academic performance. Jake's visible reaction—nodding, making eye contact, and leaning forward—indicated recognition of similar experiences. This moment marked his transition from passive attendance to active engagement.

Jake began sharing his own experiences with parental pressure, divorce-related stress, and feelings of powerlessness about family changes. Other group members responded with understanding and support, reducing Jake's isolation and increasing his investment in group participation. The identification phase continued for several weeks as Jake discovered multiple connection points with other group members.

During the exploitation phase, Jake became an active group participant who offered support and feedback to other members. He developed particular skill in helping other members identify cognitive distortions and suggested practical coping strategies. His transformation from resistant participant to group leader demonstrated Peplau's theory in action—the therapeutic relationship had enabled growth that extended far beyond his individual therapy goals.

The resolution phase required careful attention to Jake's attachment to the group and anxiety about termination. He had developed genuine friendships within the group and worried about losing this support system. We spent several sessions identifying community resources, planning ongoing contact with selected group members, and recognizing the skills he had developed that would support his continued recovery.

Case Example: Orlando's Deliberative Process During Group Crisis

During a mixed diagnostic group session focusing on coping skills, Maria, a 38-year-old with bipolar disorder, became increasingly agitated as other members discussed medication side effects. Her agitation manifested through rapid speech, fidgeting, and interrupting other speakers—behaviors that suggested emerging hypomania.

Applying Orlando's deliberative process, I first observed Maria's behavioral changes and their impact on other group members. Several members appeared uncomfortable with her interruptions, while others seemed concerned about her obvious distress. My immediate perception was that Maria's symptoms were escalating and could disrupt the therapeutic process for all members.

My thought process involved rapid assessment of several factors: Maria's current medication regimen, recent life stressors she had mentioned in previous sessions, and the group's capacity to support her while continuing their own therapeutic work. I felt concern about Maria's symptoms and responsibility to maintain therapeutic safety for all group members.

The deliberative action involved directly addressing Maria's experience while maintaining group cohesion. I paused the general discussion and said, "Maria, I notice you seem to have strong reactions to the medication discussion. Can you help us understand what you're experiencing right now?"

This intervention accomplished several goals simultaneously. It validated Maria's experience, provided her with an opportunity to express her feelings, and helped other group members understand her behavior rather than simply reacting to it. Maria explained that the medication discussion triggered fears about her own recent medication changes and concerns about symptom recurrence.

The group's response demonstrated the power of Orlando's approach—other members offered support and shared their own medication concerns, normalizing Maria's anxiety and reducing her agitation. The immediate attention to her needs prevented symptom escalation while creating a learning opportunity for all group members.

Case Example: Integrating Multiple Nursing Theories

Our PTSD support group required integration of multiple nursing theories to address the complex needs of trauma survivors. The group included eight members with diverse trauma histories—military combat, domestic violence, childhood abuse, and motor vehicle accidents—requiring flexible theoretical approaches.

Peplau's theory guided overall group development, but trauma-specific adaptations were necessary. The orientation phase extended longer than typical groups because trauma survivors often have difficulty trusting new relationships. We spent four weeks on orientation activities that emphasized safety, predictability, and member choice about participation levels.

Watson's caring theory provided additional framework for creating therapeutic environment that honored each member's dignity and inherent worth (4). This was particularly important given that trauma often involves violation of personal dignity and autonomy. Group rituals emphasized respect, shared humanity, and hope for healing.

Travelbee's human-to-human relationship model helped address the existential questions that many trauma survivors face—questions about meaning, purpose, and the nature of human relationships after betrayal or violence (5). Group discussions often explored these deeper questions rather than focusing solely on symptom management.

The integration required constant attention to individual needs within the group context. Some members needed more structure and predictability, while others benefited from flexibility and spontaneous discussions. Some members found hope through sharing their stories, while others initially needed to listen and observe before participating actively.

Success required adapting theoretical frameworks to match group needs rather than forcing group processes to fit theoretical models. The theories provided guidance and structure, but clinical judgment and member feedback determined specific interventions and group direction.

Travelbee's Human-to-Human Relationship Model

Joyce Travelbee's emphasis on human-to-human relationships rather than nurse-patient relationships offers valuable perspectives for group therapy practice. Her focus on finding meaning in suffering and developing genuine human connections aligns closely with group therapy's therapeutic factors of universality and hope.

Travelbee's theory emphasizes **rapport building** as the foundation for therapeutic relationships. In group settings, you facilitate rapport development not just between yourself and group members but among all group participants. This creates a web of supportive relationships that extends therapeutic benefits beyond the formal group sessions.

The **emerging identities** phase involves moving beyond stereotypical roles to see each person as a unique individual. Group therapy accelerates this process because members observe each other in various situations and emotional states, leading to more complete understanding of each person's humanity.

Empathy development occurs naturally in well-functioning groups as members learn to understand and respond to each other's experiences. Your role involves modeling empathetic responses and helping members develop skills in perspective-taking and emotional attunement.

The **sympathy phase** involves genuine concern for others' wellbeing that motivates helping behaviors. Group members often develop strong commitments to each other's recovery that extend beyond formal group sessions.

Rapport represents the deepest level of human connection characterized by genuine caring, mutual respect, and shared commitment to each other's growth. Groups that achieve this level of rapport often continue informal support relationships long after formal group therapy ends.

Watson's Caring Theory in Group Practice

Jean Watson's caring theory provides framework for creating group environments that honor the dignity and potential of every participant. Her emphasis on authentic presence, transpersonal caring, and healing environments directly applies to group therapy settings.

Watson's **caring moments** occur frequently in group therapy as members share vulnerable experiences and receive compassionate responses from others. Your role involves recognizing these moments and helping members appreciate their significance for healing and growth.

The **caring environment** includes both physical and emotional aspects of group settings. Physical comfort, appropriate lighting, and circle seating arrangements communicate care and respect. Emotional environment involves establishing norms of acceptance, confidentiality, and mutual support.

Transpersonal caring extends beyond individual relationships to encompass the collective spirit and energy of the group. Groups often develop their own identity and culture that reflects shared values and commitment to each other's wellbeing.

Practical Integration Strategies

Successful integration of nursing theories requires practical strategies that translate theoretical concepts into moment-to-moment group facilitation decisions. You need frameworks for assessing where individual members are in their therapeutic journeys while maintaining awareness of overall group development.

Assessment integration involves using multiple theoretical lenses to understand group member presentations and needs. A member's resistance might reflect orientation phase anxiety (Peplau), immediate needs for safety (Orlando), or search for meaning in their suffering (Travelbee).

Intervention selection draws upon various theoretical approaches depending on group needs and circumstances. Crisis situations might require Orlando's deliberative process, while termination issues might benefit from Peplau's resolution phase concepts.

Documentation should reflect theoretical frameworks used and rationale for specific interventions. This demonstrates professional nursing practice and provides foundation for supervision discussions and treatment planning.

Addressing Complex Group Dynamics

Nursing theories provide guidance for managing complex group dynamics that emerge during group therapy. Theoretical frameworks help you understand why certain dynamics develop and how to respond therapeutically rather than reactively.

Scapegoating often occurs when groups need to discharge anxiety or conflict but cannot tolerate direct confrontation. Peplau's theory suggests that scapegoating may reflect orientation phase anxiety, while Orlando's approach emphasizes immediate validation of the scapegoated member's experience.

Resistance can be understood through multiple theoretical lenses—as protection of self-identity (Travelbee), orientation phase anxiety (Peplau), or unmet immediate needs (Orlando). Understanding resistance from nursing perspectives promotes empathetic responses rather than confrontational approaches.

Group cohesion develops through application of caring theory principles, successful navigation of Peplau's phases, and responsive attention to immediate needs identified through Orlando's process.

Moving Forward with Confidence

Nursing theories provide solid foundation for group therapy practice that distinguishes your approach from other mental health disciplines. These frameworks emphasize relationship, holistic care, and the inherent dignity and potential of every individual—values that create powerful therapeutic environments.

Your theoretical knowledge must be integrated with practical skills, ongoing supervision, and continuous learning about group dynamics and therapeutic interventions. The next chapter will explore these dynamics in detail, building upon the theoretical foundation established here.

Group therapy represents an opportunity to apply nursing's unique perspectives on healing, relationship, and human potential in ways that benefit multiple individuals simultaneously. The theoretical frameworks guide your practice while clinical experience teaches you how to adapt these frameworks to meet specific group needs and circumstances.

Essential Takeaways

- Peplau's four phases (orientation, identification, exploitation, resolution) provide structure for understanding group development and individual member progress
- Orlando's deliberative nursing process offers moment-to-moment guidance for responding to group dynamics and individual needs
- Watson's caring theory creates foundation for therapeutic group environments that honor dignity and promote healing
- Travelbee's human-to-human relationship model emphasizes meaning-making and genuine connection among group members
- Theoretical integration requires flexible application based on group needs rather than rigid adherence to single frameworks
- Nursing theories distinguish group therapy practice from other disciplines through emphasis on holistic care and therapeutic relationships

Chapter 3: Group Dynamics and Therapeutic Factors

Understanding group dynamics represents the cornerstone of effective group therapy facilitation—the difference between a collection of individuals sitting in a circle and a powerful therapeutic force that transforms lives. You must develop keen observational skills to recognize the subtle interactions, unspoken alliances, and emerging patterns that shape group culture and therapeutic outcomes.

Group dynamics operate on multiple levels simultaneously, requiring your attention to both obvious interpersonal exchanges and the underlying emotional currents that drive group behavior. These dynamics can either support or hinder therapeutic progress, making your role as facilitator both challenging and tremendously rewarding.

Yalom's Therapeutic Factors in Nursing Practice

Irvin Yalom identified eleven therapeutic factors that contribute to positive group therapy outcomes, each offering unique benefits that cannot be replicated in individual therapy settings (6). These factors provide a framework for understanding how groups heal and guide your interventions to maximize therapeutic potential.

Instillation of hope occurs as group members observe others at different stages of recovery and witness real improvement over time. Unlike individual therapy where hope must be cultivated through the therapeutic relationship alone, groups provide living proof that change is possible. You facilitate this factor by highlighting member progress, celebrating small victories, and helping members recognize growth in themselves and others.

Universality represents the profound relief that comes from discovering that one's problems, feelings, and experiences are not unique or shameful. The statement "I thought I was the only one" appears frequently in group therapy as members realize their struggles are shared by others. This factor reduces isolation and shame while building connection and understanding.

Imparting information happens through both formal psychoeducation and informal sharing of coping strategies among group members. Unlike individual therapy where information flows primarily from therapist to patient, groups create multiple sources of learning as members share practical advice, resources, and hard-won wisdom about managing their conditions.

Altruism develops as group members discover their capacity to help others, which enhances self-esteem and provides sense of purpose. Members often report that helping others in the group represents their first experience of feeling useful or valuable in months or years. This factor is particularly powerful for individuals whose mental health conditions have left them feeling like burdens to others.

Corrective recapitulation of the primary family group allows members to work through family-of-origin issues within the safety of the therapy group. Members may assume familiar family roles—the caretaker, the scapegoat, the rebel—providing opportunities to recognize these patterns and develop healthier relationship dynamics.

Development of socializing techniques occurs naturally as members practice interpersonal skills within the supportive group environment. For many psychiatric patients, the group represents their primary opportunity for social interaction and skill development. You facilitate this process by modeling effective communication and providing feedback about interpersonal behaviors.

Imitative behavior allows members to try new behaviors and coping strategies observed in other group members or the facilitator. This factor accelerates learning as members experiment with different approaches to communication, problem-solving, and emotional regulation.

Interpersonal learning represents one of the most powerful therapeutic factors as members receive feedback about their impact on others and gain insight into their relationship patterns. The group serves as a social microcosm where interpersonal difficulties that exist outside the group are likely to manifest, providing opportunities for real-time intervention and skill development.

Group cohesiveness functions as the group equivalent of the therapeutic relationship in individual therapy. Cohesive groups develop strong bonds among members characterized by acceptance, support, and commitment to each other's wellbeing. This factor creates the safety necessary for members to take emotional risks and share vulnerable experiences.

Catharsis involves the expression of previously suppressed emotions within the supportive group environment. While emotional expression alone is not therapeutic, catharsis combined with cognitive insight and interpersonal feedback leads to meaningful change.

Existential factors address fundamental questions about meaning, mortality, responsibility, and isolation that underlie many psychiatric conditions. Groups provide forum for exploring these deep questions while discovering that others struggle with similar existential concerns.

Group Development Stages and Nursing Interventions

Groups progress through predictable developmental stages, each requiring different facilitation skills and interventions (7). Understanding these stages helps you anticipate challenges, normalize group experiences, and adapt your leadership style to match group needs.

Forming stage corresponds to Peplau's orientation phase, characterized by anxiety, uncertainty, and testing of boundaries. Members look to you for structure and guidance while forming initial impressions of each other. Your interventions focus on establishing safety, explaining group processes, and helping members begin to connect with each other.

During forming, members often present idealized versions of themselves while testing group rules and expectations. You provide structure through consistent facilitation style, clear communication about expectations, and warm acceptance of members' initial anxiety. Common interventions include structured introductions, explanation of group guidelines, and normalization of initial discomfort.

Storming stage involves conflict, challenging of authority, and establishment of group hierarchy. Members may compete for attention, challenge group rules, or express frustration with group processes. This stage feels uncomfortable but represents necessary development toward genuine group cohesion.

Your role during storming involves maintaining therapeutic focus while allowing appropriate expression of conflict and frustration. You model healthy conflict resolution, help members express disagreements respectfully, and prevent scapegoating or other destructive dynamics. The temptation to avoid conflict must be resisted because groups that skip storming rarely achieve genuine cohesion.

Norming stage sees establishment of group culture, shared expectations, and increased cooperation among members. The group develops its own identity and ways of operating that may differ from your initial vision but serve therapeutic purposes. Members begin taking responsibility for group functioning and supporting each other's participation.

During norming, you step back somewhat from directive leadership while remaining alert to emerging dynamics and individual needs. You reinforce positive group norms while gently redirecting problematic patterns. The group becomes more self-sustaining during this stage, requiring less active facilitation.

Performing stage represents optimal group functioning characterized by flexible roles, effective problem-solving, and genuine mutual support. Members freely express emotions, provide feedback to each other, and work actively on their therapeutic goals. The group functions as a cohesive unit while honoring individual differences and needs.

Your role during performing involves subtle facilitation that supports group functioning without interfering with natural group processes. You provide guidance when requested, offer specialized knowledge about psychiatric conditions or treatment approaches, and help members process particularly challenging material.

Adjourning stage involves preparation for group termination and consolidation of therapeutic gains. Members experience varied reactions to ending—sadness, anxiety, relief, or anger—requiring skilled facilitation to process these feelings and plan for ongoing support.

Case Example: Managing Resistance in Early Recovery Group

Our early recovery group for individuals with dual diagnosis (mental health and substance use disorders) demonstrated classic group development challenges complicated by the additional factors of addiction and psychiatric symptoms. The group included seven members in various stages of recovery from alcohol and drug use, all with co-occurring mental health conditions including depression, anxiety, and bipolar disorder.

During the initial forming stage, resistance manifested in multiple ways. Tom, a 42-year-old construction worker with alcohol use disorder and depression, attended sessions irregularly and challenged the relevance of group therapy for his problems. "I need a job, not therapy," became his frequent refrain, expressing skepticism about addressing emotional issues when practical problems felt more pressing.

Jennifer, a 29-year-old with cocaine use disorder and bipolar disorder, attended consistently but participated minimally, often stating she was "fine" and didn't need the group's help. Her resistance took the form of emotional withdrawal and insistence that her problems were different from other members' experiences.

My initial interventions focused on normalizing resistance while maintaining group structure and therapeutic focus. Rather than confronting resistance directly, I acknowledged that group therapy felt uncomfortable for most people and validated members' skepticism about treatment approaches they hadn't chosen for themselves.

The storming stage emerged around week four when Tom challenged Jennifer's claim that she was "fine," pointing out that someone who was fine wouldn't need to be in treatment. This confrontation triggered defensive responses from several members and led to heated discussion about honesty, judgment, and the right to privacy about personal struggles.

My facilitation during this conflict involved several simultaneous interventions. I validated Tom's concern about honesty in the group while also acknowledging Jennifer's right to share at her own pace. I helped the group explore different perspectives on what constitutes progress and recovery, normalizing the various approaches people take to addressing their problems.

The conflict became a turning point for group development. Jennifer acknowledged that her insistence on being "fine" reflected fear of being judged, while Tom recognized that his challenges to other members sometimes masked his own discomfort with vulnerability. Other group members shared similar struggles with balancing honesty and self-protection.

Through the norming stage, the group developed guidelines about feedback and confrontation that honored both honesty and respect. Members agreed to express concerns directly but gently, to ask permission before offering advice, and to acknowledge their own struggles when confronting others about denial or minimization.

The performing stage saw remarkable transformation in group dynamics. Tom became one of the most supportive group members, offering practical advice about employment while also addressing emotional aspects of recovery. Jennifer developed skills in expressing her feelings and asking for support, leading to better management of her bipolar symptoms and reduced substance use.

Case Example: Facilitating Therapeutic Factors in Trauma Group

Our trauma-focused group for women survivors of domestic violence demonstrated how therapeutic factors develop and interact to create powerful healing experiences. The group included six women ranging in age from 24 to 51, all in various stages of leaving abusive relationships and dealing with PTSD symptoms.

The instillation of hope factor emerged gradually as group members observed each other's progress over time. During early sessions, several members expressed doubt about their ability to ever feel safe or trust others again. Maria, who had been in the group for eight weeks when new members joined, became a living example of recovery as she shared her progress in developing new relationships and managing trauma symptoms.

Universality manifested powerfully during the third week when Linda shared her experience of hypervigilance—constantly scanning for threats and feeling unable to relax even in safe environments. The visible relief on other members' faces as they recognized similar experiences was palpable. "I thought I was going crazy," became a common refrain as members discovered that their trauma responses were normal reactions to abnormal situations.

Altruism developed as members began supporting each other through practical challenges—attending court hearings together, sharing resources about safe housing, and providing emotional support during difficult days. Sarah, who had been reluctant to share her own experiences, found her voice when supporting another member through a custody battle, discovering that helping others enhanced her own sense of empowerment.

The corrective recapitulation of family dynamics occurred as members explored how their families of origin had prepared them for abusive relationships or, conversely, how their experiences with healthy family relationships helped them recognize abuse. The group became a "family" that modeled healthy relationship dynamics—direct communication, respect for boundaries, and support without judgment.

Development of socializing techniques was particularly important for group members who had been isolated during abusive relationships. Many had lost friends and family connections, making the group their primary source of social interaction. Members practiced setting boundaries, expressing needs directly, and maintaining friendships—skills that had been dangerous in their abusive relationships but were essential for healthy connections.

Interpersonal learning occurred as members gave each other feedback about their interactions within the group. When one member consistently apologized for expressing her opinions, others gently pointed out this pattern and helped her recognize how it related to her experiences in her abusive relationship. These insights led to practice in expressing opinions without apology.

Group cohesiveness developed strongly as members formed bonds based on shared experience and mutual support. The group developed rituals—checking in about safety at the beginning of each session, celebrating members' achievements, and providing special support during particularly difficult times such as court dates or contact with former partners.

Case Example: Crisis Management During Group Conflict

During our mixed diagnostic outpatient group, a significant conflict emerged between two members that threatened group cohesion and therapeutic progress. The conflict began when James, a 35-year-old with anxiety and depression, repeatedly interrupted and gave advice to other group members without being asked. Carol, a 48-year-old with PTSD, felt triggered by his behavior because it reminded her of her controlling ex-husband.

The situation escalated during week six when Carol directly confronted James about his interruptions, stating that his behavior made her feel unsafe in the group. James responded defensively, arguing that he was only trying to help and that Carol was overreacting. Other group members appeared uncomfortable with the conflict, with some supporting each member privately after the session.

My immediate intervention focused on slowing down the interaction and helping both members express their feelings without attacking each other. I acknowledged that both members had valid concerns—James's desire to help was genuine, while Carol's need for safety was legitimate. I helped them separate current group dynamics from past experiences while also recognizing how past experiences influenced present reactions.

The conflict required several sessions to resolve and provided learning opportunities for all group members. We explored how different communication styles affect others, how past trauma can influence present interactions, and how to express needs and boundaries respectfully. James learned to ask before offering advice and to notice when his anxiety drove him to try to fix other people's problems. Carol practiced expressing her needs directly rather than enduring discomfort until it became overwhelming.

The resolution strengthened group cohesion because members learned they could disagree and work through conflicts while maintaining respect and caring for each other. The group developed new norms about giving advice, checking before offering suggestions, and expressing discomfort before it escalated to crisis levels.

Creating Psychological Safety

Psychological safety represents the foundation for all therapeutic work in group settings—the sense that one can express thoughts, feelings, and vulnerabilities without fear of judgment, rejection, or retaliation. Creating this safety requires consistent attention to group norms, facilitation style, and individual member needs.

Physical environment contributes to psychological safety through comfortable seating arranged in a circle, appropriate lighting, privacy from interruptions, and consistent meeting space. Members need to feel physically safe before they can risk emotional vulnerability.

Confidentiality agreements must be clearly explained and regularly reinforced. While you cannot guarantee that members will maintain confidentiality, you can establish clear expectations and discuss the importance of respecting each other's privacy.

Ground rules should address respect for different perspectives, prohibition of violence or threats, expectation of regular attendance, and guidelines for providing feedback to other members. These rules create predictability and structure that supports emotional safety.

Facilitator modeling demonstrates acceptance, empathy, and respect for all group members regardless of their presentations or behaviors. Your consistent therapeutic responses teach members how to interact supportively with each other.

Norm development occurs gradually as the group establishes its own culture and expectations. You can influence norm development by reinforcing positive interactions, gently redirecting problematic behaviors, and discussing group processes openly.

Managing Challenging Dynamics

Certain group dynamics require particular attention and skilled intervention to prevent them from undermining therapeutic progress. Understanding these dynamics helps you recognize early warning signs and implement appropriate interventions.

Scapegoating occurs when the group displaces anger, frustration, or anxiety onto one member who becomes the target of criticism or blame. This dynamic often reflects the group's discomfort with difficult emotions or unwillingness to address real issues. Your intervention involves protecting the scapegoated member while helping the group explore what they are avoiding through this behavior.

Monopolizing happens when one member consistently dominates group time through excessive talking, storytelling, or help-seeking behavior. While this member may have legitimate needs, their behavior prevents others from participating and can create resentment. Interventions include setting time limits, redirecting to other members, and exploring the monopolizer's anxiety about silence or sharing attention.

Silent members present different challenges because their lack of participation can indicate various issues—anxiety, depression, cultural factors, or feeling overwhelmed by more verbal members. You must balance respect for different participation styles with encouragement to engage. Interventions include direct but gentle invitations to participate, smaller group activities, and private check-ins about barriers to participation.

Subgrouping involves formation of alliances or cliques within the larger group that can create exclusion and interfere with group cohesion. Some subgrouping is natural and healthy, but problematic patterns require attention. Interventions focus on exploring the purpose of subgroups and helping all members feel included in group processes.

Measuring Group Effectiveness

Evaluation of group dynamics and therapeutic factors requires both formal assessment tools and ongoing clinical observation. You need methods to track group development, identify problematic dynamics early, and measure therapeutic outcomes.

Group Climate Inventory measures member perceptions of engagement, avoidance, and conflict within the group (8). Regular administration helps track changes in group atmosphere and identify areas needing attention.

Therapeutic Factors Scale evaluates which of Yalom's factors members find most helpful, allowing you to emphasize effective interventions and address underdeveloped factors (9).

Session Rating Scales provide immediate feedback about group members' experiences of individual sessions, helping you adjust facilitation style and group focus in real time.

Observational measures include tracking attendance patterns, participation levels, emotional expression, and interpersonal interactions. These observations provide rich information about group development and individual progress.

Building Your Skills

Effective group facilitation requires ongoing skill development and regular supervision. You must learn to track multiple individuals simultaneously while managing group-as-a-whole dynamics—a complex skill that develops through practice and reflection.

Supervision provides opportunity to process challenging group situations, explore countertransference reactions, and develop intervention strategies. Regular supervision is essential for safe and effective group practice.

Continuing education keeps you current with group therapy research and techniques. Professional conferences, workshops, and specialized training programs expand your knowledge and skills.

Personal therapy or group experience helps you understand group processes from the member perspective, increasing your empathy and effectiveness as a facilitator.

Group dynamics represent the invisible force that transforms a collection of individuals into a healing community. Your understanding of these dynamics—combined with skilled facilitation and genuine care for group members—creates the conditions for therapeutic change that extends far beyond what any individual could achieve alone.

The patterns you observe in groups reflect broader human needs for connection, understanding, and growth. By creating safe spaces for authentic relationships to develop, you facilitate healing that ripples outward into members' families, workplaces, and communities.

Core Insights for Practice

- Yalom's eleven therapeutic factors provide framework for understanding and facilitating group healing processes
- Group development stages require different facilitation approaches and interventions from forming through adjourning
- Psychological safety forms the foundation for all therapeutic work and requires consistent attention to environment, norms, and facilitation style
- Challenging dynamics such as scapegoating, monopolizing, and subgrouping require early recognition and skilled intervention
- Regular assessment of group climate and therapeutic factors guides intervention strategies and demonstrates effectiveness
- Ongoing supervision and continuing education support skill development and safe practice in group facilitation

Chapter 4: Cognitive Behavioral Therapy (CBT) Groups for Nurses

The structured approach of cognitive behavioral therapy transforms beautifully into group settings, offering psychiatric nurses a powerful framework for addressing the thinking patterns and behaviors that keep patients trapped in cycles of distress. Unlike insight-oriented therapies that focus primarily on understanding the past, CBT groups concentrate on practical skills that members can apply immediately to change their present circumstances and future outcomes.

You bring unique advantages to CBT group facilitation through your medical knowledge, assessment skills, and understanding of how psychiatric medications interact with cognitive and behavioral interventions. Your ability to recognize when physical symptoms masquerade as psychological distress—and vice versa—adds depth to CBT applications that purely psychological approaches cannot match.

Core CBT Principles for Group Application

Cognitive behavioral therapy rests on the fundamental principle that thoughts, feelings, and behaviors interconnect in patterns that either support or undermine mental health. In group settings, this principle becomes even more powerful because members can observe these connections in real-time through their interactions with each other (10).

The cognitive triangle serves as the foundation for all CBT group work. Thoughts influence feelings, which drive behaviors, which then reinforce thoughts—creating cycles that can spiral either toward wellness or distress. Group members can identify these patterns more easily in others before recognizing them in themselves, making peer feedback invaluable for developing self-awareness.

Collaborative empiricism transforms the therapist-patient relationship from expert-client to partners in investigation. In groups, this collaboration expands to include all members as investigators of their own and each other's thought patterns and behavioral choices. Members learn to question assumptions, test hypotheses about their beliefs, and gather evidence for and against their automatic thoughts.

Homework and between-session practice become group commitments rather than individual assignments. Members support each other in completing thought records, behavioral experiments, and skill practice, creating accountability and mutual encouragement that enhances compliance with therapeutic activities.

Problem-solving focus addresses specific, current difficulties rather than exploring historical or abstract issues. Groups provide multiple perspectives on problems and generate more creative solutions than individual therapy can offer. The diversity of experiences and coping strategies within groups enriches the problem-solving process.

Skill-building emphasis ensures that members learn concrete techniques they can use independently after group completion. Skills practiced in group settings feel more natural and less artificial than those learned in individual therapy because they develop through real interpersonal interactions.

Thought Records Adapted for Groups

Traditional thought records capture automatic thoughts, emotions, and behavioral responses to specific situations. Group adaptations of this fundamental CBT tool add peer feedback, multiple perspectives, and real-time processing that accelerate learning and insight development.

Shared thought records involve group members working together to complete thought records about situations that arise during group sessions. This process demystifies the technique while providing immediate examples of how thoughts influence emotions and behaviors. Members observe the thought record process before attempting their own independent records.

Peer review of thought records allows members to examine each other's thinking patterns and offer alternative perspectives. This peer feedback often proves more acceptable than facilitator suggestions because it comes from individuals facing similar challenges. Members feel less judged and more understood when peers point out cognitive distortions.

Group brainstorming for alternative thoughts generates multiple options for challenging negative automatic thoughts. Rather than struggling alone to find balanced thinking, members benefit from collective creativity and diverse viewpoints that expand their repertoire of cognitive responses.

The **round-robin technique** involves each member sharing one automatic thought while others suggest alternative perspectives. This structured approach ensures all members participate while learning from each other's situations and solutions. The technique builds group cohesion while practicing cognitive restructuring skills.

Homework review sessions dedicate group time to examining members' thought records from the previous week. These sessions reinforce learning, troubleshoot difficulties with the technique, and celebrate successes in identifying and challenging negative thinking patterns.

Case Example: Thought Record Group for Depression

Our 12-week CBT group for individuals with major depressive disorder demonstrated the power of group thought record work through the transformation of eight members who initially struggled with overwhelming negative thinking patterns. The group included individuals ranging from first-episode depression to treatment-resistant cases, creating opportunities for peer mentoring and hope inspiration.

Marcus, a 29-year-old graduate student, entered the group convinced that his depression resulted from realistic assessment of his failures rather than distorted thinking. His automatic thoughts centered on themes of inadequacy—"I'm not smart enough for graduate school," "I'll never finish my dissertation," "I'm a disappointment to my family." These thoughts triggered intense sadness and hopelessness that led to procrastination and avoidance behaviors.

During week three, the group worked on a shared thought record examining Marcus's reaction to receiving feedback on a dissertation chapter. His automatic thought—"My advisor thinks I'm incompetent"—based on suggestions for revision led to feelings of shame and behaviors including avoiding his advisor's office and postponing scheduled meetings.

Group members challenged Marcus's interpretation by exploring alternative explanations for his advisor's feedback. Sarah, a 34-year-old teacher in the group, pointed out that revision suggestions indicated investment in his success rather than judgment of his incompetence. James, a 42-year-old accountant, shared similar experiences with receiving feedback in his profession and how he had learned to view criticism as professional development rather than personal attack.

The peer feedback proved more persuasive than any facilitator intervention could have been. Marcus began to question his automatic interpretation and consider evidence for alternative thoughts such as "My advisor wants to help me succeed" and "Revision is a normal part of the writing process." These balanced thoughts reduced his emotional distress and led to behavioral changes including resuming regular advisor meetings.

As Marcus practiced thought records throughout the group, his peers continued providing feedback and support. Group members noticed patterns in his thinking—tendency to personalize professional feedback, all-or-nothing thinking about his abilities, and mind-reading assumptions about others' opinions. The group feedback helped Marcus develop a comprehensive understanding of his cognitive patterns that individual therapy had not achieved.

By group completion, Marcus had developed robust skills in identifying and challenging negative automatic thoughts. More importantly, he had internalized the group's supportive voices and could generate alternative perspectives independently. His depression scores improved significantly, and he completed his dissertation within six months of group termination.

Cognitive Restructuring Exercises

Cognitive restructuring goes beyond simple positive thinking to examine evidence for and against automatic thoughts, consider alternative explanations, and develop balanced perspectives that account for both strengths and challenges (11). Group settings accelerate this process through peer feedback and multiple viewpoints.

The evidence examination technique involves members working together to evaluate evidence supporting and contradicting negative automatic thoughts. Groups generate more thorough evidence lists than individuals working alone because different members notice different aspects of situations and bring varied life experiences to the evaluation process.

Devil's advocate exercises assign group members to argue for alternative interpretations of situations, even if they don't initially believe these alternatives. This technique helps members practice flexible thinking while discovering that multiple valid interpretations exist for most situations.

Best friend technique asks members to consider what they would tell their best friend facing the same situation. This perspective shift often reveals the harsh self-criticism and double standards that characterize depressive and anxious thinking patterns. Group members provide external validation for the gentler, more balanced perspectives.

Cognitive distortion identification games help members recognize common thinking errors through fun, interactive exercises. Groups create lists of cognitive distortions they observe in themselves and others, developing shared vocabulary for discussing thinking patterns and mutual support for challenging distorted thoughts.

Perspective-taking exercises involve members role-playing different viewpoints on problematic situations. This technique builds empathy while demonstrating how the same situation can be interpreted multiple ways depending on one's perspective and mood state.

Behavioral Activation Planning

Behavioral activation addresses the behavioral component of depression and anxiety by scheduling pleasant and meaningful activities that counteract withdrawal and avoidance patterns. Group planning adds accountability, social support, and creative brainstorming that individual behavioral activation cannot provide.

Activity brainstorming sessions generate extensive lists of potential pleasant activities by combining all group members' interests and ideas. These sessions often introduce members to new activities they had not considered and provide options for shared activities between group members.

Values clarification exercises help members identify what matters most to them as individuals, providing foundation for selecting meaningful activities rather than just pleasant ones. Group discussions about values reduce isolation and help members recognize that their core values remain intact despite their psychiatric symptoms.

Graded task assignments break overwhelming activities into manageable steps with group input and support. Members help each other identify realistic starting points and incremental goals that build confidence and momentum toward larger objectives.

Activity scheduling becomes a group project with members supporting each other's commitments and checking in about progress. This peer accountability often proves more motivating than facilitator reminders because it involves genuine concern from individuals facing similar challenges.

Problem-solving obstacles to activity engagement becomes a group process where members brainstorm solutions to common barriers such as low energy, financial constraints, transportation issues, or social anxiety about participating in activities.

Case Example: Behavioral Activation for Anxiety Group

Our anxiety management group discovered that avoidance behaviors—while providing temporary relief—ultimately increased anxiety and reduced quality of life. The eight-member group included individuals with generalized anxiety disorder, social anxiety, and panic disorder, all of whom had developed extensive avoidance patterns that limited their functioning.

Jennifer, a 26-year-old marketing professional, had stopped attending social events, declined work presentations, and avoided driving on highways following a series of panic attacks. Her world had shrunk to a few "safe" activities and locations, leaving her feeling isolated and depressed in addition to anxious.

The group's behavioral activation work began with values clarification exercises that helped Jennifer reconnect with what mattered most to her—creativity, friendship, professional growth, and adventure. She realized that her avoidance behaviors directly contradicted these core values, creating additional distress beyond her anxiety symptoms.

Group brainstorming sessions generated creative ideas for gradually expanding Jennifer's activities while managing her anxiety. Members suggested starting with brief social interactions, practicing presentation skills in low-stakes situations, and taking short highway drives during off-peak times when traffic was lighter.

The accountability aspect proved crucial for Jennifer's progress. Group members checked in weekly about her behavioral experiments, celebrated small successes, and problem-solved obstacles together. When Jennifer successfully gave a presentation at work, the group's celebration felt more meaningful than individual therapy acknowledgment because these peers understood the magnitude of her achievement.

Other group members benefited from Jennifer's courage in facing her fears. Her willingness to take risks despite feeling anxious inspired others to attempt their own behavioral experiments. The group developed a culture of encouraging appropriate risk-taking while supporting each other through the discomfort of facing feared situations.

By group completion, Jennifer had resumed most of her previous activities and added new ones that reflected her values and interests. Her anxiety symptoms decreased significantly as she learned that avoiding anxiety often increases it, while facing fears gradually reduces their power over behavior choices.

Case Example: Problem-Solving Skills Training

Our mixed diagnostic group tackled problem-solving skills when several members expressed feeling overwhelmed by life challenges that seemed impossible to address. The group included individuals with depression, anxiety, and bipolar disorder, all struggling with practical problems compounded by their psychiatric symptoms.

Robert, a 35-year-old construction worker with depression, faced multiple concurrent stressors—unemployment following a job-related injury, financial difficulties, marital conflict, and chronic pain that limited his work options. He felt paralyzed by the complexity of his situation and unable to identify where to begin addressing his problems.

The group implemented systematic problem-solving training that broke overwhelming situations into manageable components. The first step involved clearly defining specific problems rather than viewing everything as one insurmountable crisis. Robert's "impossible situation" became five distinct problems—finding suitable work, managing chronic pain, improving communication with his wife, reducing expenses, and accessing financial assistance.

Brainstorming solutions became a group exercise where all members contributed ideas for addressing Robert's employment situation. The diverse group included a teacher, a nurse, a retired mechanic, and a college student, each bringing different perspectives and knowledge about resources and opportunities. This brainstorming generated options that Robert had not considered.

Evaluating solutions involved group discussion about the pros and cons of different approaches. Members helped Robert assess the feasibility, costs, and potential benefits of various options, leading to more realistic decision-making than he could achieve while feeling depressed and overwhelmed.

Implementation planning included specific steps, timelines, and accountability measures developed with group input and support. Rather than attempting to address all problems simultaneously, Robert chose to focus initially on pain management and job training, with group members providing encouragement and practical assistance.

The group's support extended beyond formal sessions. Members shared job leads, accompanied Robert to appointments, and provided emotional support during setbacks. This practical assistance demonstrated caring while building Robert's confidence in his ability to manage life challenges.

Other group members learned problem-solving skills through participating in Robert's situation and then applying similar techniques to their own challenges. The systematic approach reduced the overwhelm that many psychiatric patients experience when facing multiple life stressors simultaneously.

Nursing-Specific CBT Adaptations

Your nursing background provides unique advantages for adapting CBT techniques to psychiatric populations. Your medical knowledge, understanding of medication effects, and holistic assessment skills create opportunities for CBT adaptations that other mental health professionals cannot provide.

Medication adherence CBT addresses the cognitive and behavioral factors that influence compliance with psychiatric medications. Thought records can identify negative beliefs about medications, while behavioral experiments can test these beliefs against actual experiences. Group members support each other through side effect management and medication adjustments.

Sleep hygiene CBT combines behavioral interventions with cognitive techniques to address sleep disturbances common in psychiatric conditions. Groups provide accountability for sleep schedule changes while addressing catastrophic thoughts about insomnia that often worsen sleep difficulties.

Pain management CBT adapts techniques for patients whose psychiatric symptoms coexist with chronic pain conditions. Thought records can identify pain catastrophizing, while behavioral activation can increase functioning despite pain. Your nursing knowledge helps distinguish physical from psychological factors affecting pain perception.

Medical procedure anxiety CBT prepares patients for medical procedures through cognitive restructuring of catastrophic thoughts and behavioral techniques for anxiety management. Groups provide opportunities to practice coping skills and learn from others' experiences with medical procedures.

Chronic illness adaptation CBT addresses the psychological impact of chronic medical conditions through cognitive restructuring of illness-related thoughts and behavioral activation despite physical limitations. Your nursing perspective helps integrate medical and psychological aspects of chronic illness management.

Documentation Templates and Progress Tracking

Systematic documentation of CBT group interventions demonstrates progress, guides treatment planning, and meets regulatory requirements while providing data for quality improvement initiatives (12). Your nursing documentation skills translate well to CBT-specific record-keeping needs.

Session documentation templates should capture group attendance, topics covered, CBT techniques used, individual member participation, homework assignments, and plans for subsequent sessions. These templates ensure consistent documentation while reducing time spent on record-keeping.

Individual progress tracking monitors each member's development of CBT skills, completion of homework assignments, symptom changes, and goal achievement. Regular assessment using standardized instruments provides objective measures of improvement that complement clinical observations.

Homework compliance tracking documents members' completion of thought records, behavioral experiments, and skill practice assignments. This data helps identify barriers to homework completion and guides modifications to improve engagement with between-session activities.

Outcome measurement should include both symptom-specific measures and functional assessment tools that capture the practical impact of CBT skill development. Pre- and post-group comparisons demonstrate treatment effectiveness while identifying areas needing additional attention.

Critical incident documentation captures significant events such as crisis situations, therapeutic breakthroughs, or group dynamic issues that affect treatment progress. These records provide valuable information for supervision discussions and treatment planning modifications.

Building CBT Group Facilitation Skills

Effective CBT group facilitation requires specific knowledge and skills that build upon your general nursing competencies. Ongoing training and supervision support skill development while ensuring safe and effective group practice.

CBT training programs provide foundation knowledge about cognitive behavioral theory, specific techniques, and group applications. Many programs offer certification credentials that demonstrate competency in CBT approaches.

Supervision arrangements should include both group process supervision and CBT-specific guidance. Experienced CBT practitioners can provide valuable feedback about technique implementation and group management strategies.

Personal CBT experience helps you understand the techniques from the client perspective, increasing empathy and effectiveness as a group facilitator. Consider participating in CBT groups or individual therapy to gain firsthand knowledge of the approach.

Outcome tracking provides feedback about your effectiveness as a CBT group facilitator and identifies areas for skill development. Regular review of group outcomes guides continuing education priorities and supervision discussions.

Preparing for Advanced Applications

As your CBT group facilitation skills develop, you may want to pursue specialized applications for specific populations or conditions. Advanced training opens opportunities for more complex group work and expanded professional roles.

Trauma-focused CBT groups require additional training in trauma-informed approaches and specific techniques for processing traumatic memories. These groups can provide powerful healing experiences but require specialized knowledge and skills.

Adolescent CBT groups need developmental adaptations that account for cognitive, emotional, and social factors unique to teenage populations. These groups often incorporate creative elements and peer influence strategies.

Geriatric CBT groups address age-related factors such as cognitive changes, chronic illness, loss and grief, and social isolation that affect older adults' mental health. These groups may require modifications for sensory impairments and shorter attention spans.

Chronic illness CBT groups focus on psychological adaptation to medical conditions and their treatment. Your nursing background provides excellent preparation for leading these specialized groups.

Looking Ahead

CBT groups provide structured, evidence-based interventions that complement your nursing knowledge and skills while offering proven techniques for addressing common psychiatric conditions. The skills you develop through CBT group facilitation will benefit your patients while expanding your professional capabilities.

The systematic approach of CBT aligns well with nursing's emphasis on assessment, planning, implementation, and evaluation. Your ability to integrate medical and psychological factors creates unique advantages in adapting CBT techniques for complex psychiatric presentations.

Practice-Ready Skills

- CBT group facilitation builds upon core nursing competencies while requiring specific training in cognitive behavioral techniques and group applications
- Thought records adapted for groups accelerate learning through peer feedback and multiple perspectives on thinking patterns
- Behavioral activation planning becomes more effective through group accountability and creative brainstorming of activity options
- Problem-solving skills training addresses the overwhelming nature of multiple life stressors common in psychiatric populations
- Nursing-specific adaptations integrate medical knowledge with CBT techniques for comprehensive patient care
- Documentation and outcome tracking demonstrate treatment effectiveness while supporting quality improvement initiatives

Chapter 5: Dialectical Behavior Therapy (DBT) Skills Groups

The intense emotions and behavioral challenges that characterize many psychiatric conditions require specialized interventions that go beyond traditional cognitive approaches. Dialectical Behavior Therapy skills groups offer psychiatric nurses powerful tools for helping patients develop concrete skills for managing emotional crises, improving relationships, and building lives worth living despite ongoing mental health challenges.

DBT groups differ fundamentally from traditional therapy groups—they function more like classes where members learn specific skills through instruction, practice, and homework assignments. You serve as teacher and coach rather than traditional group therapist, providing psychoeducation about skills while helping members adapt techniques to their individual circumstances and treatment goals.

Understanding the DBT Framework

Dialectical Behavior Therapy emerged from Marsha Linehan's work with individuals diagnosed with borderline personality disorder who had not responded to traditional therapeutic approaches (13). The "dialectical" component emphasizes balance—accepting current reality while working toward change, validating emotions while learning to regulate them, and maintaining individual identity while building healthy relationships.

Biosocial theory explains how emotional dysregulation develops through the interaction of biological vulnerabilities and invalidating environments. This framework helps both you and group members understand that emotional sensitivity is not a character flaw but a legitimate medical condition requiring specific skills and treatments.

Four modules structure provides systematic skill development across domains that research has identified as most problematic for individuals with emotional dysregulation. Each module builds upon previous learning while targeting specific aspects of emotional and behavioral functioning.

Skills-focused approach distinguishes DBT groups from process-oriented therapy groups. Members attend to learn concrete techniques rather than process relationships or explore underlying issues. This structure works particularly well for individuals who feel overwhelmed by emotional intensity and need practical tools before they can engage in deeper therapeutic work.

Homework emphasis requires members to practice skills between sessions and track their use of techniques in daily life. This between-session practice is essential for skill generalization and long-term improvement in emotional regulation and interpersonal functioning.

Mindfulness Skills Module

Mindfulness forms the foundation for all other DBT skills by teaching present-moment awareness and non-judgmental acceptance of internal experiences. These skills help patients step back from emotional intensity and respond thoughtfully rather than react impulsively to challenging situations (14).

Wise mind concept teaches the balance between emotional mind (driven by feelings) and reasonable mind (focused on logic and facts). Wise mind integrates both emotional and rational information to make decisions that align with long-term goals and values rather than momentary impulses.

The **STOP technique** provides immediate crisis intervention tool: Stop what you're doing, Take a breath, Observe your thoughts and feelings, and Proceed with awareness. This simple technique interrupts impulsive responses and creates space for thoughtful decision-making during emotional crises.

Observe skills teach patients to notice their thoughts, emotions, and sensations without immediately acting on them. This observational stance reduces the intensity of difficult emotions and prevents impulsive behaviors that often worsen situations.

Describe skills involve putting experiences into words without adding interpretations or judgments. This technique helps patients gain clarity about what is actually happening versus what they think or fear might be happening.

Participate skills encourage full engagement in activities without self-consciousness or divided attention. This mindful participation increases enjoyment and effectiveness while reducing rumination and worry about past or future events.

Non-judgmental stance involves observing experiences without labeling them as good or bad, right or wrong. This acceptance reduces the secondary emotional reactions (shame about feeling angry, anxiety about being depressed) that often intensify psychiatric symptoms.

Case Example: Mindfulness Skills with Trauma Survivors

Our DBT skills group for women with trauma histories demonstrated how mindfulness techniques can be adapted for individuals whose hypervigilance and dissociation make traditional meditation approaches challenging or potentially harmful. The eight-member group included survivors of childhood abuse, domestic violence, and sexual assault, all struggling with PTSD symptoms and emotional dysregulation.

Amanda, a 31-year-old nurse with childhood sexual abuse history, initially found mindfulness exercises triggering because focusing inward increased her awareness of trauma-related body sensations and intrusive memories. Her attempts at meditation led to panic attacks and dissociative episodes that left her feeling more distressed than before the exercises.

We adapted mindfulness techniques to accommodate trauma responses by starting with eyes-open exercises that maintained connection to external reality. Amanda learned to practice mindfulness while engaging in simple activities like coloring, walking, or organizing objects—activities that provided enough structure to prevent dissociation while building present-moment awareness.

The group discovered that mindfulness could be practiced during routine nursing tasks—taking vital signs, charting, and patient care activities. This revelation helped Amanda integrate mindfulness into her daily work life without requiring additional time or triggering trauma responses. She learned to use mindful breathing during stressful patient situations and practiced the STOP technique between patient encounters.

Other group members benefited from Amanda's adaptations and contributed their own modifications based on their trauma responses and life circumstances. Maria, a domestic violence survivor, practiced mindfulness while cooking because the kitchen had become a safe space after leaving her abusive relationship. Jennifer used mindful walking in her garden as a way to reconnect with her body in a positive way.

The group's collective wisdom about trauma-informed mindfulness exceeded what any individual could have developed alone. Members learned to recognize early warning signs of dissociation, develop grounding techniques that worked for their specific trauma responses, and adapt traditional mindfulness exercises to accommodate their unique needs and triggers.

By module completion, Amanda had developed a personalized mindfulness practice that enhanced her emotional regulation without triggering trauma responses. She reported feeling more present during social interactions, less overwhelmed by work stress, and better able to enjoy positive experiences without anxiety about when they might end.

Distress Tolerance Skills Module

Distress tolerance skills address the reality that painful emotions are part of human experience and cannot always be eliminated or avoided. These skills help patients survive crisis situations without making them worse through impulsive or self-destructive behaviors (15).

Crisis survival skills provide immediate techniques for managing intense emotions without engaging in behaviors that create additional problems. These skills acknowledge that sometimes the goal is simply surviving difficult moments rather than fixing or changing the situation.

TIPP technique offers rapid nervous system regulation through Temperature change (cold water on face or ice cubes), Intense exercise, Paced breathing, and Progressive muscle relaxation. These physiological interventions can rapidly reduce emotional intensity during crisis situations.

Distraction skills help patients redirect attention away from overwhelming emotions or urges until the intensity naturally decreases. Effective distractions require full engagement and may include physical activities, mental exercises, emotional experiences, or social connections.

Self-soothing techniques involve nurturing oneself through difficult emotions using the five senses—comforting sights, sounds, smells, tastes, and textures. These skills counteract the self-criticism and emotional harshness that often accompany psychiatric conditions.

Improving the moment focuses on making unbearable situations slightly more bearable through techniques like visualization, prayer or meditation, encouragement, and finding meaning in suffering. These skills acknowledge that some situations cannot be changed but responses to them can be modified.

Pros and cons analysis helps patients make decisions during emotional crises by examining both short-term and long-term consequences of different behavioral choices. This technique slows down decision-making and reduces impulsive actions that often worsen situations.

Radical acceptance involves accepting reality as it is without approving of it or giving up efforts to create change. This skill reduces the additional suffering that comes from fighting against unchangeable situations while preserving energy for areas where change is possible.

Emotion Regulation Skills Module

Emotion regulation skills teach patients how to understand, experience, and modify emotions in healthy ways rather than being overwhelmed or controlled by emotional experiences (16). These skills are particularly valuable for individuals whose psychiatric conditions involve mood instability or emotional intensity.

Emotion identification helps patients recognize and name their emotional experiences accurately. Many individuals with psychiatric conditions have difficulty distinguishing between different emotions or identifying the triggers that precipitate emotional responses.

Function of emotions education teaches that emotions serve important purposes—they provide information about situations, motivate action, and communicate needs to others. Understanding emotional functions reduces shame about having feelings while building motivation to regulate emotions effectively.

Opposite action involves acting opposite to emotional urges when the emotion is not justified by facts or when acting on the emotion would be ineffective or harmful. This technique helps patients break cycles of avoidance, aggression, or other emotion-driven behaviors that maintain or worsen their difficulties.

Mastery activities build confidence and positive emotions through engaging in activities that provide sense of accomplishment or competence. These activities counteract depression and build resilience for managing future emotional challenges.

Pleasant activities scheduling ensures regular positive experiences that improve mood and provide motivation for continuing recovery efforts. This technique addresses the anhedonia (inability to experience pleasure) common in depression and other psychiatric conditions.

PLEASE skills maintain emotional vulnerability through Physical illness treatment, balanced Eating, avoiding mood-Altering substances, balanced Sleep, and Exercise. These basic self-care practices create foundation for emotional stability and reduce susceptibility to mood fluctuations.

Case Example: Emotion Regulation with Bipolar Disorder

Our DBT skills group for individuals with bipolar disorder focused heavily on emotion regulation techniques because mood episodes often begin with subtle emotional changes that can be addressed through early intervention. The six-member group included individuals with Bipolar I, Bipolar II, and cyclothymic disorder, all struggling with mood instability despite medication treatment.

Carlos, a 28-year-old teacher with Bipolar I disorder, experienced frequent mood episodes despite stable medication regimen because he had not learned to recognize early warning signs or implement behavioral interventions that could prevent full episodes. His mood changes felt sudden and overwhelming, leading to impulsive decisions that created additional problems during both manic and depressive periods.

The group's work on emotion identification helped Carlos recognize the subtle physical and cognitive changes that preceded mood episodes. He learned to track his mood daily using standardized rating scales and identify patterns related to sleep, stress, and seasonal changes that influenced his emotional stability.

Opposite action skills proved particularly valuable for Carlos during developing depressive episodes. When he noticed early signs of depression—decreased energy, pessimistic thoughts, and social withdrawal urges—he practiced opposite actions including increasing social contact, engaging in physical activity, and maintaining normal sleep schedules even though these actions felt difficult.

During early hypomanic episodes, opposite action involved slowing down rather than increasing activity, avoiding major decisions, and seeking input from trusted friends or family members who could provide reality testing about his judgment and behavior. These techniques helped prevent progression to full manic episodes that had previously resulted in hospitalization.

The group provided accountability and support for Carlos's mood monitoring and early intervention efforts. Other members helped him recognize warning signs he might miss and celebrated his successes in preventing mood episodes through skillful behavior choices.

PLEASE skills became a group focus because all members needed better self-care habits to maintain mood stability. The group developed strategies for regular sleep schedules, stress management, and avoiding substances that could trigger mood episodes. Members supported each other through challenges like social events involving alcohol or work situations that disrupted sleep patterns.

By skills group completion, Carlos had experienced his longest period of mood stability since his initial diagnosis. He had successfully used DBT skills to prevent three potential mood episodes and felt confident in his ability to manage bipolar disorder as a chronic condition rather than being at its mercy.

Interpersonal Effectiveness Skills Module

Interpersonal effectiveness skills help patients build and maintain healthy relationships while managing the social challenges that often accompany psychiatric conditions (17). These skills address communication patterns, boundary setting, and conflict resolution that support recovery and improve quality of life.

DEAR MAN technique provides structure for asking for what you need or saying no to requests: Describe the situation, Express feelings, Assert needs, Reinforce benefits, stay Mindful of goals, Appear confident, and Negotiate when possible. This framework reduces anxiety about difficult conversations while increasing effectiveness in getting needs met.

GIVE skills maintain relationships during disagreements or conflicts: be Gentle in approach, show Interest in the other person's perspective, Validate their feelings and viewpoints, and use Easy manner that keeps interactions light when possible. These skills prevent relationship damage during necessary but difficult conversations.

FAST skills preserve self-respect during interpersonal interactions: be Fair to yourself and others, avoid Apologies when not warranted, Stick to your values, and be Truthful about your feelings and needs. These skills address the tendency many psychiatric patients have to sacrifice their own needs to maintain relationships.

Relationship building skills focus on developing new connections and strengthening existing relationships through positive interactions, shared activities, and mutual support. These skills are particularly important for patients whose psychiatric conditions have damaged or limited their social networks.

Conflict resolution techniques provide frameworks for addressing disagreements constructively rather than avoiding conflict or engaging in destructive arguments. These skills help patients navigate inevitable relationship challenges without damaging important connections.

Case Example: Interpersonal Skills with Social Anxiety

Our DBT skills group for individuals with social anxiety disorder demonstrated how interpersonal effectiveness skills can address both the symptoms of anxiety and the social isolation that often results from avoidance behaviors. The seven-member group included individuals with generalized social anxiety, specific social phobias, and social anxiety secondary to other psychiatric conditions.

Rachel, a 25-year-old graduate student, had developed severe social anxiety following a series of panic attacks during class presentations. Her avoidance of social situations had led to academic difficulties, loss of friendships, and increasing depression that complicated her anxiety symptoms.

DEAR MAN skills helped Rachel communicate with professors about her anxiety without feeling ashamed or making excuses for her difficulties. She learned to describe her situation factually, express her commitment to academic success, assert her need for accommodations, and reinforce the benefits of working together to address her challenges.

The group practiced DEAR MAN through role-playing exercises that allowed Rachel to build confidence before attempting real-world applications. Group members provided feedback about her communication style and suggested modifications that might increase her effectiveness while maintaining her authenticity.

GIVE skills helped Rachel maintain relationships with classmates and friends who had become frustrated with her frequent cancellations and avoidance of social activities. She learned to validate their disappointment while gently explaining her challenges and showing genuine interest in maintaining their friendships.

Rachel discovered that many people responded positively to honest communication about her anxiety rather than the vague excuses she had been making. Friends appreciated understanding the real reasons for her behavior and often offered support and accommodations she hadn't expected.

FAST skills addressed Rachel's tendency to over-apologize and minimize her own needs in social situations. She practiced sticking to her values about academic excellence while being truthful about her anxiety rather than pretending everything was fine when it wasn't.

The group setting provided a safe place for Rachel to practice interpersonal skills with peers who understood social anxiety from personal experience. Group members offered realistic feedback about social interactions and supported each other through the discomfort of gradually increasing social contact.

By skills group completion, Rachel had returned to regular class attendance, re-established several friendships, and developed confidence in her ability to navigate social situations despite ongoing anxiety. She had learned that avoiding social anxiety often increases it, while facing it with appropriate skills reduces its impact on her life.

Nursing Adaptations for Inpatient Settings

Inpatient psychiatric settings require modifications to standard DBT skills group protocols because of shorter lengths of stay, acute symptom presentations, and the intensity of the hospital environment. Your nursing knowledge of inpatient dynamics and medical factors affecting psychiatric presentations allows for effective adaptations.

Shortened modules focus on essential skills that can be learned and applied during brief hospitalizations. Priority skills include crisis survival techniques, basic emotion regulation, and simple interpersonal effectiveness strategies that support discharge planning and outpatient follow-up.

Medical integration considers how medications, medical conditions, and physical symptoms affect patients' ability to learn and apply DBT skills. You can adapt techniques for patients with cognitive impairment, adjust expectations for individuals experiencing medication side effects, and integrate skills with medical treatment plans.

Crisis stabilization focus emphasizes skills most relevant for managing acute psychiatric symptoms and preventing readmission. These skills help patients survive immediate crises while building foundation for longer-term outpatient DBT participation.

Nursing care plan integration connects DBT skills with individualized treatment goals and nursing interventions. Skills practice becomes part of routine nursing care rather than additional programming that competes with medical treatment priorities.

Discharge planning preparation uses DBT skills to address challenges patients anticipate facing after hospitalization. Skills practice can focus on medication adherence, follow-up appointment attendance, and crisis management in community settings.

Outcome Measurement and Progress Tracking

Systematic measurement of DBT skills group outcomes provides data about treatment effectiveness while identifying areas where individual members need additional support or different interventions. Your nursing assessment skills support accurate and meaningful outcome measurement.

Skills use tracking monitors how frequently members apply DBT techniques in daily life and which skills they find most helpful for their specific challenges. This information guides ongoing treatment planning and helps identify skills that need additional practice or modification.

Symptom measurement using standardized instruments provides objective data about changes in emotional regulation, interpersonal functioning, and overall psychiatric symptoms. Regular assessment helps distinguish between normal fluctuations and significant improvement or deterioration.

Functional assessment measures improvements in daily living skills, social functioning, and quality of life that result from DBT skills application. These functional improvements often continue developing after symptom improvement plateaus.

Crisis behavior tracking documents changes in frequency and severity of self-harm, substance use, impulsive behaviors, and other crisis situations that DBT skills are designed to address. Reduction in these behaviors indicates successful skills acquisition and application.

Building Toward Advanced Practice

DBT skills group facilitation provides excellent foundation for advanced psychiatric nursing practice and specialized interventions. Your experience with these intensive skill-building groups prepares you for leadership roles in complex treatment programs.

Individual DBT therapy requires additional training but builds naturally on skills group experience. The combination of individual therapy and skills groups provides the most effective DBT treatment for complex presentations.

DBT program development involves creating systematic programs that integrate skills groups with other treatment modalities. Your nursing knowledge supports program development that addresses both psychiatric and medical needs.

Training and supervision of other nurses in DBT approaches expands access to these effective interventions while advancing your own professional development and expertise in evidence-based treatments.

Sustainable Practice

The intensive nature of DBT skills groups requires attention to your own self-care and professional development to maintain effectiveness and prevent burnout. The same skills you teach group members can support your own emotional regulation and stress management.

Regular supervision provides essential support for managing challenging group dynamics and complex patient presentations. DBT-informed supervision includes attention to both technical skills and the emotional impact of working with individuals experiencing severe emotional dysregulation.

Continuing education in DBT approaches keeps you current with research findings and technique refinements while building toward advanced certification credentials that expand professional opportunities.

Foundational Insights

- DBT skills groups function as educational classes rather than traditional therapy groups, requiring clear structure and systematic skill instruction
- Four modules (mindfulness, distress tolerance, emotion regulation, interpersonal effectiveness) address core areas of difficulty for individuals with emotional dysregulation
- Trauma-informed adaptations ensure that mindfulness and other techniques remain safe and beneficial for survivors of abuse and violence
- Inpatient modifications focus on crisis stabilization and essential skills that can be learned during brief hospitalizations
- Outcome measurement tracks both skill use and functional improvements that result from DBT techniques application
- Integration with nursing care plans and medical treatment enhances overall patient outcomes while supporting discharge planning and community follow-up

Chapter 6: Mindfulness and Stress Reduction Groups

The ancient practice of mindfulness meets modern psychiatric nursing in groups that teach patients to develop a different relationship with their thoughts, emotions, and physical sensations. Rather than being overwhelmed by internal experiences or fighting against them, group members learn to observe their mental and physical processes with curiosity and acceptance while developing skills for responding thoughtfully rather than reacting automatically to challenging situations.

Your nursing background provides unique advantages for leading mindfulness groups because you understand how stress affects both mental and physical health, how medications influence patients' ability to concentrate and relax, and how to adapt techniques for individuals with various psychiatric conditions and cognitive abilities. You bring medical knowledge to contemplative practices, creating safe and effective interventions for vulnerable populations.

Evidence Base for Mindfulness in Psychiatric Nursing

Research demonstrates significant benefits of mindfulness-based interventions for multiple psychiatric conditions, making these approaches valuable additions to standard nursing care (18). Studies consistently show improvements in anxiety, depression, chronic pain, and overall quality of life among individuals who participate in structured mindfulness programs.

Neurobiological research reveals that mindfulness practice creates measurable changes in brain structure and function, particularly in areas responsible for emotional regulation, attention, and stress response. These changes provide biological foundation for the clinical improvements observed in mindfulness practitioners.

Meta-analyses of mindfulness interventions show effect sizes comparable to established psychiatric treatments, with particularly strong results for anxiety disorders, depression, and chronic pain conditions. The evidence supports mindfulness as both standalone intervention and complement to medication and psychotherapy.

Long-term follow-up studies indicate that benefits of mindfulness training continue developing after formal instruction ends, suggesting that patients learn skills they can use independently to maintain and improve their mental health over time.

Healthcare utilization research shows that patients who participate in mindfulness programs use fewer emergency services, require fewer hospitalizations, and report greater satisfaction with their overall healthcare experience. These findings support mindfulness as cost-effective intervention that improves outcomes while reducing healthcare costs.

Progressive Muscle Relaxation Scripts

Progressive muscle relaxation teaches patients to recognize and release physical tension while developing awareness of the mind-body connection that influences both physical and emotional well-being. This technique works particularly well for individuals with anxiety disorders, trauma histories, or chronic pain conditions.

Basic PMR sequence involves systematically tensing and releasing muscle groups throughout the body while paying careful attention to the contrast between tension and relaxation. Start with feet and legs, progress through abdomen and chest, then arms and hands, finishing with neck and facial muscles.

Shortened versions accommodate patients with limited attention spans, physical limitations, or time constraints. Five-minute PMR focuses on major muscle groups—legs, abdomen, arms, shoulders, and face—providing significant benefits in shorter timeframe suitable for busy schedules or acute care settings.

Trauma-informed modifications ensure safety for individuals whose hypervigilance or dissociation makes standard PMR potentially triggering. Keep eyes open, maintain awareness of surroundings, use gentler muscle contractions, and emphasize choice about participation level throughout the exercise.

Pain-adapted techniques modify PMR for individuals with chronic pain conditions who cannot safely tense certain muscle groups. Focus on areas without pain, use visualization of tension and release rather than actual muscle contraction, and emphasize breathing and mental relaxation components.

Group PMR sessions create shared relaxation experiences that build group cohesion while teaching individual skills. Members often report feeling more connected to others after sharing relaxation experiences, and group setting provides motivation for practice that individual instruction may lack.

Case Example: Progressive Muscle Relaxation for Chronic Pain Group

Our chronic pain support group included eight individuals with various pain conditions—fibromyalgia, arthritis, chronic back pain, and neuropathy—all struggling with the emotional impact of persistent physical discomfort. Traditional relaxation techniques often proved challenging because tensing muscles increased pain rather than providing relief.

Margaret, a 58-year-old retired teacher with fibromyalgia, initially resisted PMR because previous attempts had triggered pain flares that lasted for days. Her fibromyalgia made her muscles hypersensitive to tension, and traditional PMR instructions to "tighten muscles as much as possible" caused significant distress rather than relaxation.

We developed modified PMR protocols that emphasized mental awareness of muscle states rather than physical manipulation. Margaret learned to notice areas of existing tension and practice "letting go" rather than creating additional tension through muscle contractions. This approach honored her body's limitations while still providing benefits of increased body awareness.

Visualization-based PMR became Margaret's preferred technique. She learned to imagine tension flowing out of her body like water, visualize muscles softening and lengthening, and use breathing to support the relaxation process. These mental techniques provided many of the same benefits as traditional PMR without triggering pain responses.

The group setting proved crucial for Margaret's success with modified PMR. Other members shared their own adaptations for various physical limitations, creating a repertoire of techniques that accommodated different types of pain and disability. Group members validated each other's need for modifications rather than viewing them as failure to do the technique "correctly."

Breathing integration enhanced PMR effectiveness for Margaret and other group members. Deep, slow breathing patterns activated the parasympathetic nervous system, providing physiological relaxation that complemented the mental aspects of tension release. Group members learned to use breathing as anchor during PMR when physical discomfort made concentration difficult.

Regular practice with group support led to significant improvements in Margaret's pain management and overall well-being. She reported better sleep quality, reduced anxiety about pain episodes, and increased confidence in her ability to manage fibromyalgia symptoms through self-care techniques rather than relying solely on medication.

Other group members benefited from Margaret's courage in requesting modifications and her willingness to share what worked for her specific condition. The group developed a culture of adaptation and creativity that honored individual differences while maintaining focus on relaxation and stress reduction goals.

Guided Imagery Exercises

Guided imagery uses imagination and visualization to create mental experiences that promote relaxation, healing, and positive emotional states. These techniques work particularly well for patients who have difficulty with body-focused mindfulness practices or who respond better to creative and imaginative interventions.

Safe place visualization helps patients create internal refuge they can access during times of stress or crisis. This basic imagery exercise builds skills in self-soothing while providing concrete technique for managing anxiety and overwhelming emotions.

Healing imagery focuses mental attention on areas of physical or emotional pain with intention of promoting recovery and comfort. While not claiming to cure medical conditions, healing imagery can reduce stress that complicates recovery and enhance patients' sense of participation in their healing process.

Future self visualization helps patients imagine themselves successfully managing their psychiatric conditions and achieving their recovery goals. This technique builds hope and motivation while providing mental rehearsal for desired behavioral changes.

Sensory-rich scenarios engage multiple senses to create vivid mental experiences that feel real and meaningful to participants. Effective imagery includes visual details, sounds, smells, textures, and even tastes that make the imagined experience as engaging as possible.

Nature-based imagery draws upon the calming effects of natural environments to promote relaxation and restoration. These exercises work well for patients who have limited access to outdoor spaces or who live in urban environments with minimal nature contact.

Breathing Techniques for Anxiety

Breathing practices offer immediate and accessible tools for managing anxiety symptoms while building foundation for other mindfulness techniques. These practices can be used discreetly in any situation, making them particularly valuable for patients who experience anxiety in social or work settings.

Box breathing involves equal counts for inhalation, hold, exhalation, and hold—typically four counts each. This structured breathing pattern interrupts anxiety responses while providing simple focus for anxious minds that tend toward worry and rumination.

4-7-8 breathing extends exhalation longer than inhalation—inhale for 4 counts, hold for 7, exhale for 8. The extended exhalation activates parasympathetic nervous system responses that counteract anxiety and promote relaxation.

Belly breathing emphasizes diaphragmatic breathing rather than shallow chest breathing that often accompanies anxiety. Teaching patients to breathe into their abdomen rather than upper chest provides more efficient oxygenation while triggering relaxation responses.

Counted breathing involves simply counting breaths from one to ten and starting over, providing gentle focus that occupies the mind without requiring complex concentration. This technique works well for patients with attention difficulties or severe anxiety who cannot manage more complex practices.

Breathing with visualization combines breath awareness with imagery—imagining breathing in calm or light and breathing out tension or darkness. This combination engages both cognitive and physiological relaxation mechanisms for enhanced effectiveness.

Case Example: Breathing Techniques for Panic Disorder

Our anxiety disorders group included five individuals with panic disorder who struggled with sudden, intense episodes of fear accompanied by physical symptoms that felt life-threatening. Traditional breathing exercises often felt impossible during panic attacks, requiring modifications that could be used during acute symptoms.

David, a 32-year-old accountant, experienced panic attacks several times weekly, often during important meetings or social events. His attempts to control his breathing during attacks typically worsened his symptoms because focusing on breathing made him more aware of feeling short of breath and increased his fear of suffocation.

We developed **crisis breathing techniques** that could be used during panic attacks without requiring perfect execution or creating additional pressure. David learned to focus on making his exhales longer than his inhales without counting or timing—simply emphasizing the out-breath to activate calming physiological responses.

Recovery breathing provided techniques for the period after panic attacks when David felt exhausted and shaky. These gentle breathing practices helped restore normal physiological functioning and reduce anticipatory anxiety about future attacks. Recovery breathing emphasized comfort and self-care rather than perfect technique.

The group setting allowed David to practice breathing techniques while experiencing manageable levels of anxiety, building confidence in his ability to use these tools when needed. Group members practiced together during anxiety-provoking discussions, learning to apply breathing skills in real-time rather than only during calm moments.

Portable breathing techniques could be used discreetly in any situation without drawing attention to David's anxiety management efforts. He learned to use bathroom breaks for brief breathing exercises, practice breathing techniques while walking between meetings, and integrate mindful breathing into routine activities.

Other group members contributed their own discoveries about breathing during anxiety, creating a collection of techniques that addressed different situations and symptom presentations. Some members found counting helpful while others preferred visualization; some needed structure while others benefited from flexibility.

Group support reduced David's shame about having panic attacks and increased his willingness to use breathing techniques consistently rather than only during crises. The shared understanding that anxiety is a medical condition requiring skillful management—rather than a personal weakness—supported his commitment to practice.

Case Example: Walking Meditation for Depression Group

Our depression recovery group discovered that traditional sitting meditation often increased rumination and negative thinking rather than providing relief from depressive symptoms. The physical movement and sensory engagement of walking meditation proved more effective for group members struggling with low energy and persistent negative thoughts.

Sandra, a 45-year-old social worker with recurrent major depression, found that sitting quietly with her thoughts typically led to rumination about past mistakes and future concerns rather than present-moment awareness. Her mind seemed to use meditation time as opportunity for worry and self-criticism rather than relaxation and acceptance.

Mindful walking provided gentle physical activity that improved mood while teaching mindfulness skills through movement rather than stillness. Sandra learned to focus attention on the physical sensations of walking—feeling feet contact the ground, noticing changes in balance and weight distribution, observing how muscles coordinated to create forward movement.

Outdoor walking meditation combined mindfulness with nature exposure and light therapy, addressing multiple factors that contribute to depression. Group members walked together in nearby parks, practicing mindfulness techniques while benefiting from fresh air, natural light, and gentle exercise that research shows improves mood.

Sensory awareness walking engaged multiple senses to create rich, present-moment experiences that interrupted depressive rumination. Sandra learned to notice sounds around her, observe visual details in her environment, feel air temperature and breeze, and even notice smells during outdoor walking sessions.

The group structure provided motivation for Sandra to participate in walking meditation even when depression made her want to isolate and remain inactive. Group members supported each other through low-energy days and celebrated small improvements in mood and energy that resulted from regular practice.

Indoor walking adaptations made practice possible during weather limitations or for group members with mobility restrictions. These adaptations included walking in hallways, focusing on very slow, deliberate movement, and emphasizing quality of attention rather than distance covered or speed of walking.

Integration with activity scheduling connected walking meditation with behavioral activation approaches to depression treatment. Sandra learned to use mindful walking as bridge between periods of inactivity and more demanding daily activities, building momentum for greater engagement with her recovery goals.

Safety Considerations for Dissociative Disorders

Mindfulness practices can be triggering for individuals with dissociative disorders, requiring careful modifications that maintain therapeutic benefits while ensuring emotional and psychological safety. Your nursing assessment skills help identify patients who need trauma-informed mindfulness adaptations.

Grounding techniques should be taught before introducing mindfulness practices for patients with dissociation histories. These techniques help patients maintain connection to present reality when internal focus triggers dissociative responses.

Eyes-open practices maintain visual connection to external environment, reducing risk of dissociation that can occur when patients close their eyes and focus internally. Many mindfulness benefits can be achieved through practices that maintain environmental awareness.

Choice and control must be emphasized throughout mindfulness instruction, allowing patients to modify or discontinue practices if they become triggering. Patients need permission to adapt techniques to their safety needs rather than following instructions that feel dangerous.

Shorter practices reduce risk of dissociation that can develop during extended periods of internal focus. Five to ten-minute practices may be more appropriate than traditional twenty to thirty-minute sessions for patients with dissociation vulnerabilities.

Movement-based alternatives provide mindfulness benefits through physical activity rather than internal focus. Walking meditation, gentle yoga, or mindful daily activities may be safer options for patients with severe dissociation histories.

Integration with Medication Management

Mindfulness practices complement psychiatric medications while providing skills that enhance treatment compliance and reduce reliance on crisis interventions. Your nursing knowledge supports effective integration of contemplative practices with medical treatment approaches.

Medication mindfulness teaches patients to pay attention to their medication experiences—noticing side effects, observing therapeutic benefits, and developing awareness of how medications affect their physical and emotional states. This awareness supports informed collaboration with prescribers about medication adjustments.

Timing considerations account for how psychiatric medications affect patients' ability to concentrate and participate in mindfulness practices. Some medications may cause sedation that makes meditation difficult, while others may improve focus and emotional regulation that supports mindfulness development.

Side effect management uses mindfulness techniques to cope with uncomfortable medication side effects while maintaining compliance with prescribed treatments. Breathing techniques can reduce nausea, progressive muscle relaxation can address muscle tension, and mindfulness can help patients tolerate temporary discomfort for long-term benefits.

Transition support applies mindfulness skills during medication changes, which often involve temporary symptom fluctuations that challenge patients' coping abilities. Mindfulness provides stable resource during medication adjustments that can feel destabilizing.

Building Sustainable Practice

Long-term benefits of mindfulness require ongoing practice that continues after formal group instruction ends. Your role includes helping patients develop realistic practice routines that fit their lifestyles while maintaining motivation for continued skill development.

Informal mindfulness integrates present-moment awareness into daily activities rather than requiring separate meditation time. Patients learn to practice mindfulness while eating, showering, washing dishes, or walking—activities they already do that can become opportunities for mindfulness development.

Technology supports including meditation apps, online guided practices, and reminder systems help patients maintain practice consistency while providing variety and progression in their mindfulness development.

Community connections through meditation groups, mindfulness meetups, or ongoing practice groups provide social support and motivation for continued practice. Many patients benefit from community involvement that extends beyond formal treatment settings.

Progress tracking helps patients recognize subtle improvements in attention, emotional regulation, and stress management that result from mindfulness practice. Regular self-assessment maintains motivation during periods when progress feels slow or unclear.

Wisdom for Practice

Mindfulness groups offer psychiatric nurses opportunity to share ancient wisdom through modern therapeutic applications that address both mental and physical aspects of suffering. Your medical knowledge and clinical skills create unique foundation for adapting contemplative practices to serve individuals with serious mental health conditions.

The simplicity of mindfulness practices can be deceptive—learning to pay attention to present-moment experience without judgment requires patience, practice, and skilled guidance that honors both the power and potential risks of these approaches. Your nursing presence provides safety and support that allows vulnerable individuals to explore internal experiences that may have felt threatening or overwhelming.

Essential Learning Elements

- Evidence-based mindfulness interventions show effectiveness comparable to established psychiatric treatments while providing skills patients can use independently
- Progressive muscle relaxation requires modifications for patients with chronic pain, trauma histories, or physical limitations that make standard techniques inappropriate
- Guided imagery provides alternative approach for patients who struggle with body-focused mindfulness practices or who respond better to creative interventions
- Breathing techniques offer immediate anxiety management tools that can be used discreetly in any situation
- Safety considerations for dissociative disorders require trauma-informed modifications that maintain benefits while preventing triggering responses
- Integration with medication management enhances treatment compliance while providing skills that complement pharmacological interventions

Chapter 7: Psychopharmacology Education Groups

The complexity of psychiatric medications challenges both patients and healthcare providers, yet many individuals receive prescriptions with minimal education about how these powerful substances work, what to expect, and how to manage the inevitable side effects that accompany most psychotropic treatments. Medication education groups bridge this knowledge gap while creating supportive communities where patients can share experiences, learn from each other, and develop realistic expectations about their pharmaceutical treatments.

Your nursing expertise uniquely positions you to lead these educational groups because you understand both the clinical pharmacology of psychiatric medications and the practical realities patients face when taking them daily. You see patients throughout their medication journeys—from initial prescriptions through adjustments, side effects, and long-term maintenance—providing perspective that purely clinical or academic approaches cannot match.

Patient Medication Education Groups Framework

The structured approach of Patient Medication Education Groups (PMEGs) provides systematic framework for delivering medication education that improves knowledge, adherence, and satisfaction with psychiatric treatment (19). This evidence-based model transforms medication education from one-time prescriber consultation into ongoing educational process supported by peer learning and professional guidance.

Educational rather than therapeutic focus distinguishes PMEGs from traditional therapy groups. Members attend to learn specific information about medications rather than to process emotions or work through interpersonal issues. This educational focus appeals to patients who want practical information but may resist traditional therapy approaches.

Structured curriculum ensures consistent delivery of essential medication information while allowing flexibility to address group-specific questions and concerns. The systematic approach covers fundamental topics all patients need while providing opportunities to explore issues particularly relevant to specific group compositions.

Peer learning components harness the collective wisdom of individuals who have experience with various medications, side effects, and management strategies. Patients often trust peer experiences more than professional recommendations, making group learning particularly powerful for medication acceptance and adherence.

Professional guidance from nurses ensures accurate information delivery while providing medical perspective on medication questions that arise during group discussions. Your nursing knowledge helps distinguish between common side effects that can be managed and serious reactions requiring immediate medical attention.

Homework assignments reinforce learning through practical applications such as tracking side effects, researching specific medications, or developing personal medication management systems. These assignments bridge the gap between group learning and daily medication practices.

Understanding Psychiatric Medications Module

The foundation module addresses basic pharmacology concepts in accessible language that empowers patients to become informed participants in their medication treatment rather than passive recipients of prescriptions they don't understand.

Medication categories education helps patients understand why they've been prescribed specific types of medications and how different drug classes address various psychiatric symptoms. Understanding the logic behind medication choices reduces anxiety and increases cooperation with treatment recommendations.

Brain chemistry basics explains in simple terms how psychiatric conditions affect neurotransmitter function and how medications work to correct these imbalances. This scientific foundation reduces stigma by framing mental illness as medical condition requiring medical treatment rather than personal weakness requiring willpower.

Onset expectations prepare patients for the reality that most psychiatric medications require weeks or months to achieve full therapeutic effects. This education prevents premature discontinuation when patients don't experience immediate improvement and helps maintain hope during initial treatment periods.

Individual variation factors explain why medications affect different people differently and why finding the right medication often requires trying several options. This education reduces frustration with the trial-and-error process and helps patients understand that medication adjustments reflect normal medical practice rather than treatment failure.

Combination approaches educate patients about why multiple medications are sometimes necessary and how different drugs can work together synergistically. This education addresses common concerns about "taking too many pills" and helps patients understand complex treatment regimens.

Case Example: Antidepressant Education for First-Episode Depression

Our depression medication education group included eight individuals newly diagnosed with major depressive disorder, most receiving their first psychiatric medications. The group's primary goal was reducing anxiety about starting antidepressants while building realistic expectations about treatment timelines and potential side effects.

Maria, a 34-year-old teacher, exemplified common concerns about starting psychiatric medication. She worried that taking antidepressants meant she was "weak" or "crazy," feared becoming dependent on medication, and expected immediate relief from her depressive symptoms. Her misconceptions about antidepressants created resistance to treatment that threatened her recovery.

The **brain chemistry education** proved transformative for Maria's understanding of depression and its treatment. Learning that depression involves measurable changes in neurotransmitter function—similar to how diabetes involves insulin dysfunction—reframed her condition as legitimate medical illness requiring appropriate medical treatment.

Visual aids showing normal versus depressed brain functioning helped Maria understand why she couldn't simply "think her way out" of depression and why medication was necessary to restore normal brain chemistry. This scientific foundation reduced her shame about needing medication while building confidence in her treatment approach.

Onset education prepared Maria for the reality that antidepressants typically require four to six weeks to show significant effects and may take months to achieve full benefits. This timeline education prevented disappointment when she didn't feel better after the first week and maintained her commitment to treatment during the initial adjustment period.

Group discussions about **individual variation** helped Maria understand why her medication choice might differ from friends' prescriptions and why dose adjustments were normal rather than concerning. Hearing other group members' experiences with different antidepressants normalized the process of finding the right medication and dose.

The **side effect education** prepared Maria for common initial side effects such as nausea, headaches, and sleep changes while teaching her which effects were temporary versus those requiring medical attention. This preparation reduced anxiety about normal side effects while emphasizing the importance of communicating with her prescriber about concerning symptoms.

Maria's transformation from reluctant medication recipient to informed treatment participant demonstrated the power of education in building treatment alliance and improving outcomes. She completed the full course of treatment, experienced significant improvement in her depression, and became an advocate for medication education among her friends and colleagues.

Side Effect Management Strategies Module

Side effects represent the primary reason patients discontinue psychiatric medications, yet many of these effects can be managed effectively through practical strategies that allow patients to continue beneficial treatments (20). Education about side effect management transforms obstacles into manageable challenges.

Common side effects overview prepares patients for effects they're likely to experience while distinguishing between normal, temporary reactions and serious problems requiring immediate medical attention. This education reduces anxiety about expected effects while emphasizing appropriate caution about dangerous reactions.

Timing strategies teach patients how to minimize side effects through careful attention to when and how they take medications. Simple adjustments such as taking sedating medications at bedtime or taking stomach-irritating drugs with food can dramatically improve tolerability.

Lifestyle modifications address side effects through changes in diet, exercise, sleep habits, and daily routines that complement medication effects while reducing unwanted reactions. These modifications often provide additional mental health benefits beyond side effect management.

Communication templates give patients language for discussing side effects with prescribers, including how to describe symptoms accurately and advocate for appropriate treatment modifications. Many patients minimize or fail to report side effects due to communication difficulties rather than lack of concern.

Persistence versus switching decisions help patients evaluate when to continue medications despite side effects versus when to request changes in treatment. This decision-making education prevents both premature discontinuation and unnecessary tolerance of problematic effects.

Drug Interactions and Safety Module

Psychiatric medications can interact with other prescription drugs, over-the-counter medications, supplements, and even foods, creating potentially dangerous situations that patients must understand to maintain their safety while receiving effective treatment.

Prescription drug interactions education covers the most common and serious interactions between psychiatric medications and other prescription drugs. Patients learn to always inform all healthcare providers about their psychiatric medications and to check with prescribers before starting new medications.

Over-the-counter considerations address interactions with common medications such as pain relievers, cold medicines, and sleep aids that patients might not consider problematic. Many over-the-counter drugs can interfere with psychiatric medication effectiveness or increase side effects.

Supplement interactions cover vitamins, herbs, and nutritional supplements that can affect psychiatric medication function. St. John's wort, for example, can reduce the effectiveness of many psychiatric medications, while certain vitamins can increase side effects.

Food and beverage interactions explain how alcohol, caffeine, and certain foods can interact with psychiatric medications. Patients learn about timing considerations for taking medications with meals and which substances to avoid entirely.

Emergency preparedness teaches patients how to communicate their medication information during medical emergencies and what information to carry with them. This education can be life-saving during crisis situations when patients cannot advocate for themselves.

Case Example: Mood Stabilizer Education for Bipolar Disorder

Our bipolar disorder medication group focused heavily on lithium and other mood stabilizers because these medications require more careful monitoring and patient education than many other psychiatric drugs. The eight-member group included individuals newly diagnosed with bipolar disorder and others struggling with medication adherence despite years of treatment.

Robert, a 28-year-old electrician recently diagnosed with Bipolar I disorder, felt overwhelmed by the complexity of lithium treatment and the multiple safety considerations involved. His manic episode had resulted in job loss and relationship problems, leaving him motivated for treatment but anxious about the long-term implications of taking mood stabilizers.

Lithium education covered the unique aspects of this medication, including the need for regular blood level monitoring, the narrow range between therapeutic and toxic levels, and the importance of maintaining consistent dosing and adequate hydration. Robert learned that lithium's effectiveness requires careful attention to details that other medications don't demand.

The group practiced **safety protocols** including recognizing early signs of lithium toxicity, understanding when to hold doses during illness or dehydration, and knowing which situations require immediate medical consultation. This practical safety education reduced Robert's anxiety about lithium while building confidence in his ability to take it safely.

Monitoring schedules education helped Robert understand the rationale for frequent blood tests and medical appointments during initial treatment. Learning that monitoring frequency decreases once stable levels are achieved made the initial intensive monitoring feel more manageable and temporary.

Group discussions about **lifestyle adaptations** for lithium treatment covered practical issues such as maintaining consistent sleep schedules, managing salt and fluid intake, and handling medication during travel or schedule disruptions. Other group members shared practical strategies for incorporating these considerations into daily life.

Long-term perspectives from group members who had taken lithium successfully for years provided hope and practical wisdom about living well with bipolar disorder. These peer mentors demonstrated that lithium treatment was compatible with productive, fulfilling lives while sharing honest information about ongoing challenges and management strategies.

Robert's education about mood stabilizers transformed his relationship with his diagnosis and treatment. He developed confidence in his ability to manage the complexities of lithium treatment while maintaining realistic expectations about the ongoing nature of bipolar disorder management.

Case Example: Antipsychotic Education for Schizophrenia

Our schizophrenia education group addressed the unique challenges of antipsychotic medications, which often produce more noticeable side effects than other psychiatric drugs while treating symptoms that can impair patients' insight into their need for treatment. The six-member group included individuals with schizophrenia, schizoaffective disorder, and treatment-resistant depression requiring antipsychotic augmentation.

David, a 25-year-old college student with recent onset schizophrenia, struggled with accepting his diagnosis and the need for long-term antipsychotic treatment. His cognitive symptoms made learning difficult, while his lack of insight into his illness created resistance to medication adherence that concerned his family and treatment team.

Symptom education helped David understand the relationship between his experiences—hearing voices, feeling suspicious of others, having trouble concentrating—and the brain changes that antipsychotic medications address. This education was provided in simple, concrete terms that accommodated his cognitive difficulties.

Visual aids showing brain scan differences in schizophrenia helped David's family understand his condition as medical illness rather than character flaw or poor choices. This family education reduced blame and criticism while building support for David's treatment adherence and recovery efforts.

Side effect education covered both common and serious effects of antipsychotic medications, with particular attention to movement-related side effects that can be especially concerning for young patients. David learned to recognize early signs of movement problems and understood the importance of reporting these effects promptly.

The group addressed **cognitive side effects** honestly, acknowledging that some antipsychotics can affect thinking and memory while emphasizing that untreated psychosis causes more severe cognitive impairment. This balanced presentation helped David understand the trade-offs involved in medication treatment.

Weight management education covered the metabolic effects of many antipsychotic medications and provided practical strategies for maintaining healthy weight and preventing diabetes. Group members shared successful approaches to diet and exercise that had helped them manage these common side effects.

David's gradual acceptance of his diagnosis and treatment reflected the power of peer education and support in addressing conditions that affect insight and judgment. The group provided reality testing and practical wisdom that complemented professional treatment while building David's confidence in his ability to manage his condition successfully.

Long-Acting Injectable Education Module

Long-acting injectable (LAI) medications offer significant advantages for certain patients but require specialized education to address common concerns and misconceptions about this delivery method.

Advantages of LAI treatment include guaranteed medication delivery that eliminates daily adherence decisions, more stable blood levels that may reduce side effects, and reduced burden of daily medication routines. Patients learn that LAI treatment often improves quality of life while maintaining therapeutic effectiveness.

Injection process education covers what to expect during injection appointments, including injection site rotation, potential discomfort management, and scheduling considerations. This education reduces anxiety about the injection process while building realistic expectations.

Transition planning from oral to injectable medications requires careful coordination and patient education about overlapping treatments and timeline expectations. Patients learn that switching to LAI typically involves gradual transition rather than immediate change.

Myth-busting education addresses common misconceptions about injectable medications, such as beliefs that they're only for "severe" cases or that they represent punishment for non-adherence. Education emphasizes that LAI treatment is medical choice based on individual needs and preferences.

Scheduling and logistics education helps patients plan for regular injection appointments and understand the flexibility available in timing while maintaining therapeutic effectiveness. This practical information supports successful LAI treatment implementation.

Interactive Teaching Methods

Effective medication education requires interactive approaches that engage patients actively rather than passive listening to lectures. Your nursing communication skills support creative teaching methods that accommodate diverse learning styles and cognitive abilities.

Role-playing exercises allow patients to practice discussing medications with prescribers, family members, and other healthcare providers. These exercises build communication skills while addressing anxiety about medication-related conversations.

Medication sorting activities help patients learn to categorize their medications by class, timing, and purpose. These hands-on activities reinforce learning while building practical medication management skills.

Side effect brainstorming sessions encourage patients to share experiences and management strategies while building collective wisdom about medication challenges. These discussions normalize difficulties while providing practical solutions.

Question and answer formats create opportunities for patients to voice concerns and receive accurate information in supportive group settings. Structured Q&A sessions ensure all patients can participate while addressing common concerns.

Guest speakers including pharmacists, prescribers, and experienced patients provide varied perspectives and specialized knowledge that enriches group learning. These presentations expose patients to different viewpoints while building professional relationships.

Health Literacy Adaptations

Many patients struggle with health literacy challenges that interfere with medication understanding and adherence. Your nursing assessment skills help identify these challenges and adapt education accordingly.

Language simplification involves translating medical terminology into everyday language that patients can understand and remember. Complex pharmacological concepts are explained through analogies and metaphors that relate to patients' experiences.

Visual aids including diagrams, charts, and illustrations support learning for patients who struggle with written information or prefer visual learning styles. These materials reinforce verbal education while providing reference tools for home use.

Repetition and reinforcement accommodate patients with memory difficulties or attention problems by presenting information multiple times in different formats. Key concepts are reviewed throughout the group series rather than presented only once.

Cultural adaptations consider how cultural background affects medication beliefs and practices. Education addresses cultural concerns while respecting diverse perspectives on health and healing.

Reading level considerations ensure that written materials match patients' literacy levels while maintaining accuracy and completeness. Materials are tested with patient groups to ensure comprehensibility.

Building Collaborative Relationships

Medication education groups create opportunities for building collaborative relationships between patients and healthcare providers that extend beyond the group setting to improve overall treatment quality.

Shared decision-making skills teach patients how to participate actively in medication decisions rather than passively accepting prescriber recommendations. This collaboration improves treatment satisfaction while building patient autonomy.

Advocacy training helps patients communicate effectively with prescribers about their needs, concerns, and preferences regarding medication treatment. These skills reduce power imbalances while improving therapeutic relationships.

Question preparation teaches patients how to prepare for prescriber appointments by organizing questions, tracking symptoms, and advocating for their needs. This preparation maximizes appointment effectiveness while building patient confidence.

Treatment partnership concepts emphasize that effective medication treatment requires collaboration between patients and providers rather than compliance with expert recommendations. This partnership approach improves adherence while respecting patient autonomy.

Looking Beyond the Group

The knowledge and skills patients develop through medication education groups should support their ongoing treatment and recovery long after group completion. Your role includes preparing patients for independent medication management and ongoing learning.

Building connections with pharmacy services, prescribers, and other healthcare providers creates resources patients can access for ongoing medication questions and support. These professional relationships extend group benefits beyond the formal program.

Encouraging participation in peer support groups, online communities, and advocacy organizations provides ongoing sources of medication information and support that complement professional treatment.

The medication education foundation established through these groups supports patients throughout their recovery journeys, building confidence and knowledge that improve treatment outcomes while reducing healthcare utilization and costs.

Practical Wisdom

Medication education represents one of the most concrete and immediately applicable interventions you can provide as a psychiatric nurse. The knowledge patients gain through these groups has measurable impacts on their treatment adherence, side effect management, and overall satisfaction with psychiatric care.

Your unique position as a nurse allows you to bridge the gap between prescriber expertise and patient experience, creating educational programs that honor both scientific knowledge and lived experience. This balance creates powerful learning environments that transform medication treatment from burden into tool for recovery.

Core Learning Elements

- Patient Medication Education Groups provide structured, evidence-based framework for systematic delivery of medication information in supportive group settings
- Understanding psychiatric medications module builds foundation knowledge about brain chemistry, medication categories, and realistic expectations for treatment outcomes
- Side effect management strategies transform common obstacles into manageable challenges through practical techniques and lifestyle modifications
- Drug interactions and safety education protects patients while building confidence in their ability to take medications safely
- Long-acting injectable education addresses misconceptions while highlighting advantages of this treatment delivery method
- Interactive teaching methods and health literacy adaptations ensure effective learning across diverse patient population

Chapter 8: Medication Adherence and Compliance Groups

The gap between prescribed psychiatric medications and actual patient use represents one of the most significant challenges in mental health care, with non-adherence rates reaching 50-75% across various psychiatric conditions. Medication adherence groups address this challenge through systematic exploration of barriers, peer support for problem-solving, and skill development that transforms medication-taking from daily burden into manageable aspect of recovery-oriented care.

You bring unique perspectives to adherence support because you understand both the clinical necessity of consistent medication use and the real-world challenges patients face in maintaining complex medication regimens while managing psychiatric symptoms, side effects, and competing life demands. Your nursing experience with diverse patient populations provides foundation for addressing the multiple factors that influence medication adherence decisions.

Evidence-Based Adherence Interventions

Research identifies multiple factors that influence medication adherence, requiring multifaceted interventions that address knowledge deficits, practical barriers, motivational concerns, and support system limitations (21). Effective adherence interventions combine education, behavioral strategies, social support, and ongoing monitoring to create sustainable medication-taking behaviors.

Behavioral interventions focus on establishing routines, removing barriers, and building positive associations with medication-taking behaviors. These approaches treat adherence as learned behavior that can be strengthened through reinforcement and environmental modifications.

Motivational approaches explore patients' ambivalence about medication use while building intrinsic motivation for adherence based on personal values and recovery goals. These interventions avoid confrontation while supporting patients' autonomous decision-making about their treatment.

Educational components ensure patients have accurate information about their medications while addressing misconceptions that interfere with adherence. Education alone rarely improves adherence, but it provides foundation for other intervention approaches.

Social support interventions harness family, peer, and professional relationships to support consistent medication use while reducing isolation and stigma that can undermine adherence efforts.

Technology-assisted approaches use reminder systems, monitoring apps, and digital support tools to supplement human interventions while providing convenience and privacy that many patients value.

Medication Calendars and Tracking Sheets

Visual tracking tools help patients monitor their medication use while identifying patterns that either support or undermine adherence goals. These tools provide objective data about adherence behavior while building awareness of factors that influence daily medication decisions.

Daily tracking calendars provide simple checkbox systems for recording medication use while noting factors such as mood, side effects, and significant events that might affect adherence. These calendars reveal patterns that patients might not notice without systematic tracking.

Weekly planning sheets help patients prepare for upcoming challenges to adherence such as travel, schedule changes, or stressful events. This proactive planning prevents common adherence failures while building confidence in patients' ability to maintain medication routines.

Side effect monitoring forms track the relationship between medication use and side effects, helping patients and prescribers understand patterns and make informed decisions about treatment modifications. This monitoring often reveals that side effects are less frequent or severe than patients initially perceived.

Mood tracking integration combines medication adherence monitoring with mood rating scales to help patients observe the relationship between consistent medication use and symptom improvement. This data provides powerful motivation for continued adherence.

Barrier identification sheets help patients recognize and problem-solve obstacles to consistent medication use. Common barriers include forgetting, cost concerns, side effects, complexity of regimens, and competing priorities that interfere with medication routines.

Case Example: Adherence Support for Bipolar Disorder

Our bipolar disorder adherence group included six individuals who had experienced multiple mood episodes despite having access to effective medications. The group's focus was identifying and addressing specific barriers that interfered with consistent medication use while building sustainable adherence strategies.

Jennifer, a 32-year-old marketing manager with Bipolar II disorder, struggled with medication adherence during periods of mood stability when she felt "normal" and questioned the need for continued treatment. Her pattern involved discontinuing medications during good periods, followed by depressive episodes that required intensive treatment and time off work.

Adherence tracking revealed Jennifer's pattern clearly—she maintained excellent adherence during symptomatic periods but gradually decreased consistency as she felt better. This pattern helped her recognize that feeling normal was actually a sign that her medications were working, not evidence that she no longer needed them.

Group discussions about **insight fluctuations** in bipolar disorder helped Jennifer understand that questioning medication necessity during stable periods is common and predictable rather than valid reason for discontinuation. Other group members shared similar experiences and strategies for maintaining adherence during asymptomatic periods.

Values clarification exercises helped Jennifer connect medication adherence to her career goals, relationship aspirations, and personal values. She recognized that medication consistency supported her ability to maintain employment and relationships rather than limiting her freedom as she had previously believed.

The group developed **maintenance motivation strategies** for periods when Jennifer felt well and questioned medication necessity. These strategies included reviewing past episode consequences, maintaining mood tracking even during stable periods, and scheduling regular check-ins with group members who could provide objective feedback about early warning signs.

Routine integration helped Jennifer incorporate medication-taking into established daily habits rather than treating it as separate task requiring special attention. She learned to take medications with morning coffee and evening tooth brushing, making adherence automatic rather than requiring daily decisions.

Jennifer's transformation from sporadic medication user to consistent adherent demonstrated the power of peer support and systematic barrier identification in changing adherence behavior. She maintained medication consistency for over a year following group completion and experienced her longest period of mood stability since diagnosis.

Problem-Solving Adherence Barriers

Systematic problem-solving approaches help patients address specific obstacles to medication adherence through structured analysis and creative solution development. This process transforms overwhelming adherence challenges into manageable problems with concrete solutions.

Barrier identification begins with honest assessment of factors that interfere with medication adherence, including practical obstacles, emotional concerns, and environmental challenges. Patients often discover that their adherence problems have specific, addressable causes rather than reflecting lack of motivation or commitment.

Root cause analysis explores underlying factors that contribute to apparent adherence barriers. Forgetting medications might reflect depression-related cognitive difficulties, cost concerns might mask embarrassment about financial struggles, or family conflict might underlie apparent medication resistance.

Solution brainstorming generates multiple potential approaches to identified barriers while encouraging creative thinking and peer input. Group settings provide diverse perspectives and experiences that expand solution options beyond what individuals could generate alone.

Implementation planning involves selecting specific solutions to try, establishing timelines and accountability measures, and anticipating obstacles to solution implementation. This planning bridges the gap between good intentions and actual behavior change.

Evaluation and modification tracks solution effectiveness while making adjustments based on real-world testing. This iterative process recognizes that adherence solutions often require refinement and modification to achieve lasting success.

Peer Support Strategies

Peer support harnesses the shared experience and mutual understanding among individuals facing similar medication challenges to create powerful support systems that complement professional interventions.

Buddy systems pair group members for mutual support and accountability between group sessions. These partnerships provide ongoing encouragement and problem-solving support that extends group benefits beyond formal meeting times.

Experience sharing allows group members to learn from each other's successes and failures with various adherence strategies. This sharing provides practical wisdom that complements professional recommendations while building hope and motivation.

Mentorship relationships connect newer group members with individuals who have achieved stable adherence to provide guidance, encouragement, and reality testing about recovery expectations and medication experiences.

Group problem-solving harnesses collective wisdom to address individual members' adherence challenges while building group cohesion and mutual investment in each other's success.

Celebration and recognition of adherence achievements reinforces positive behavior while building group culture that values medication consistency as important recovery milestone.

Case Example: Peer Support for Depression Treatment

Our depression medication adherence group included eight individuals struggling with antidepressant compliance despite having access to effective treatments and supportive prescribers. The group's emphasis on peer support created powerful connections that transformed members' relationships with their medications and recovery processes.

Marcus, a 45-year-old construction worker, had started and stopped multiple antidepressants over three years, usually discontinuing treatment after a few weeks due to side effects or lack of rapid improvement. His pattern of medication cycling had created frustration with treatment while preventing him from experiencing the full benefits of consistent antidepressant use.

Peer mentorship connected Marcus with James, a 52-year-old electrician who had achieved stable recovery through consistent antidepressant use after years of similar struggles. James's ability to relate to Marcus's work environment and male identity created trust that enabled honest discussion about depression and medication concerns.

James shared his own history of **medication cycling** and the breakthrough realization that he had never given any antidepressant adequate time to work. This peer wisdom carried more weight than professional recommendations because it came from someone who understood Marcus's experiences and perspective.

Accountability partnerships involved Marcus and another group member checking in weekly about medication adherence and mood changes. These check-ins provided motivation for consistency while creating early warning system for adherence problems or mood deterioration.

Group **experience sharing** revealed that many members had similar patterns of premature medication discontinuation and that achieving stable adherence often required multiple attempts and strategy modifications. This sharing normalized Marcus's struggles while building hope for eventual success.

Problem-solving sessions helped Marcus address specific barriers to adherence including morning grogginess that made him skip doses, concerns about sexual side effects affecting his marriage, and shame about needing medication to function normally. Group input provided practical solutions while reducing isolation and stigma.

Marcus's development of consistent medication use and significant improvement in depression demonstrated the power of peer relationships in supporting behavior change. His success within the group motivated other members while building his confidence as someone who could help others facing similar challenges.

Case Example: Technology Integration for Schizophrenia

Our schizophrenia medication adherence group explored technology solutions to support consistent medication use among individuals whose cognitive symptoms and complex medication regimens created significant adherence challenges. The six-member group included individuals with varying levels of technology comfort and access.

Carlos, a 28-year-old with schizoaffective disorder, struggled with medication adherence due to cognitive difficulties that affected his memory and executive functioning. His complex regimen of multiple daily medications at different times created confusion that led to missed doses and occasional dangerous double-dosing.

Smartphone app evaluation involved group members testing various medication reminder applications to identify features that were most helpful for individuals with cognitive challenges. The group discovered that simple, repetitive reminder systems worked better than complex tracking applications that required significant cognitive effort.

Carlos found success with an app that provided **audio reminders** at medication times along with simple yes/no confirmation buttons. The audio component helped overcome reading difficulties while the simple interface accommodated his attention problems and processing speed limitations.

Pill organizer systems combined traditional weekly pill organizers with technology supports such as smart pill caps that tracked opening times and sent smartphone notifications about missed doses. This hybrid approach provided visual confirmation of medication-taking while adding technological backup for memory difficulties.

Group **technology troubleshooting** sessions helped members address common problems such as forgotten phone chargers, changed medication schedules, and technical difficulties with applications. Peer support proved essential because group members understood the cognitive challenges that made technology use difficult.

Family integration involved teaching family members how to support technology-assisted adherence without creating conflict or undermining patient autonomy. Family members learned to provide backup support for technology systems while respecting patients' independence in medication management.

Carlos's successful integration of technology supports with traditional adherence strategies demonstrated that even individuals with significant cognitive challenges could benefit from carefully selected technological tools when supported by peer learning and ongoing troubleshooting assistance.

Cultural Considerations in Medication Beliefs

Cultural background significantly influences patients' beliefs about medications, illness, and appropriate treatment approaches, requiring culturally sensitive adherence interventions that respect diverse worldviews while promoting evidence-based treatment.

Cultural assessment explores patients' cultural background, traditional healing practices, family influences, and spiritual beliefs that might affect medication attitudes and adherence behavior. This assessment identifies potential conflicts between cultural beliefs and psychiatric treatment recommendations.

Belief exploration creates safe space for patients to discuss concerns about medications that might conflict with cultural or religious teachings. These discussions honor cultural diversity while providing education about medical perspectives on psychiatric treatment.

Integration strategies help patients find ways to combine psychiatric medications with cultural practices and beliefs rather than viewing them as incompatible. This integration often involves collaboration with traditional healers, religious leaders, or cultural advisors.

Family education addresses cultural factors that influence family attitudes toward psychiatric medications while building support for patient adherence goals. Family involvement respects cultural values about collective decision-making while supporting individual treatment needs.

Community resources connect patients with culturally appropriate support services and advocacy organizations that can provide ongoing assistance with adherence challenges while honoring cultural identity and values.

Family Involvement Strategies

Family members often play significant roles in supporting or undermining medication adherence, requiring targeted interventions that build family capacity for positive support while addressing problematic dynamics that interfere with adherence goals.

Family education provides accurate information about psychiatric conditions and their treatment while addressing misconceptions that might lead family members to discourage medication use. This education helps family members understand their role in supporting recovery.

Communication training teaches family members how to provide supportive encouragement for medication adherence without creating conflict or undermining patient autonomy. These skills help families balance support with respect for adult patients' independence.

Practical support strategies help families provide assistance with medication management tasks such as prescription refills, appointment transportation, and side effect monitoring while avoiding over-involvement that undermines patient self-efficacy.

Conflict resolution addresses family disagreements about medication use while helping families develop collaborative approaches to supporting adherence goals. These interventions recognize that family conflict can significantly undermine adherence efforts.

Boundary setting helps patients establish appropriate limits on family involvement in medication decisions while maintaining supportive relationships. These boundaries protect patient autonomy while preserving family connections.

Technology Integration Solutions

Modern technology offers multiple tools for supporting medication adherence, but successful implementation requires careful selection and customization based on individual patient needs, preferences, and technological capacity.

Reminder systems range from simple smartphone alarms to sophisticated applications that track medication use, send customized notifications, and provide adherence feedback. The key is matching reminder complexity to individual cognitive abilities and preferences.

Monitoring applications help patients track medication use, side effects, mood changes, and other factors that influence adherence while providing data for sharing with healthcare providers. These apps can identify patterns that might not be apparent without systematic tracking.

Virtual support groups connect patients with others facing similar adherence challenges while providing 24/7 access to peer support and information. These online communities complement in-person groups while providing ongoing support between sessions.

Telemedicine integration allows patients to discuss adherence challenges with healthcare providers through video consultations, phone calls, or secure messaging systems. This technology removes transportation barriers while providing timely support for adherence problems.

Smart pill bottles and electronic monitoring devices provide objective data about medication-taking behavior while sending reminders and alerts about missed doses. These devices can be particularly helpful for patients with memory difficulties or complex medication regimens.

Measuring Adherence Outcomes

Systematic measurement of adherence improvements provides data about intervention effectiveness while identifying patients who need additional support or different approaches to achieve adherence goals.

Self-report measures including standardized adherence questionnaires provide patient perspectives on medication-taking behavior while identifying barriers and motivations that influence adherence decisions.

Objective monitoring through pill counts, pharmacy refill data, and electronic monitoring devices provides accurate data about actual medication use that may differ from patient self-reports.

Clinical outcomes including symptom improvement, hospitalization rates, and functional status changes provide evidence about the clinical benefits of improved adherence while demonstrating the value of adherence interventions.

Quality of life measures assess how adherence improvements affect patients' overall well-being, satisfaction with treatment, and ability to achieve personal goals beyond symptom reduction.

Long-term follow-up tracks adherence sustainability after intervention completion while identifying factors that support or undermine long-term adherence maintenance.

Sustaining Motivation

Long-term medication adherence requires ongoing motivation that extends beyond initial crisis periods or acute symptoms that originally motivated treatment engagement.

Values-based motivation connects medication adherence to patients' personal values and life goals rather than relying solely on symptom improvement or external pressure from healthcare providers or family members.

Progress recognition helps patients identify and celebrate improvements that result from consistent medication use, including subtle changes that might otherwise go unnoticed.

Maintenance planning addresses the reality that motivation for adherence naturally fluctuates over time and develops strategies for maintaining consistency during periods of reduced motivation or increased life stress.

Ongoing support connections with peer groups, healthcare providers, and family members provide resources for addressing adherence challenges that arise after formal intervention completion.

Medication adherence represents both individual responsibility and community support challenge that requires ongoing attention throughout the recovery process. Your role as a nurse positions you uniquely to provide the combination of medical knowledge, practical support, and empathetic understanding that effective adherence interventions require.

The relationships and skills patients develop through adherence groups create foundation for long-term recovery that extends far beyond medication consistency to include broader self-care practices, healthcare engagement, and social support development that support overall well-being.

Key Implementation Strategies

- Evidence-based adherence interventions address multiple factors including knowledge, motivation, practical barriers, and social support through systematic approaches that treat adherence as learned behavior
- Medication tracking tools provide objective data about adherence patterns while building patient awareness of factors that influence daily medication decisions
- Systematic problem-solving transforms adherence challenges into manageable problems with concrete solutions through structured analysis and creative solution development
- Peer support strategies harness shared experience and mutual understanding to create powerful support systems that complement professional interventions
- Cultural considerations ensure that adherence interventions respect diverse worldviews while promoting evidence-based psychiatric treatment
- Technology integration provides modern tools for supporting adherence while requiring careful selection based on individual patient needs and technological capacity

Chapter 9: Adolescent Psychiatric Group Interventions

Working with adolescents in group therapy settings requires you to navigate the unique developmental challenges of a population caught between childhood and adulthood, struggling with identity formation while managing psychiatric conditions that can derail normal developmental processes. Teenagers bring energy, creativity, and capacity for rapid change to group settings, but they also present challenges that demand specialized approaches fundamentally different from adult or child interventions.

Your nursing perspective provides distinct advantages in adolescent mental health groups because you understand the biological changes occurring during puberty, the impact of psychiatric medications on developing brains, and the complex interplay between physical health and emotional well-being that characterizes this developmental stage. You also recognize that adolescent psychiatric conditions often represent the early manifestations of lifelong mental health challenges, making effective intervention during these formative years essential for long-term outcomes.

Integrated Model Combining Interpersonal and Feminist Perspectives

Adolescent group therapy benefits from theoretical frameworks that address both the relational aspects of teenage development and the power dynamics that affect young people's experiences in families, schools, and healthcare systems (22). The integration of interpersonal and feminist perspectives creates space for adolescents to explore identity formation while addressing systemic factors that contribute to their distress.

Interpersonal focus recognizes that adolescent psychiatric symptoms often emerge in the context of relationship difficulties with peers, family members, or romantic partners. Group settings provide natural laboratories for practicing interpersonal skills while receiving feedback from age-matched peers who understand the social pressures of adolescence.

Feminist perspectives address power imbalances that affect adolescents, particularly regarding their limited autonomy in treatment decisions, educational settings, and family systems. These approaches validate teenagers' experiences of powerlessness while building skills for advocacy and empowerment within existing systems.

Identity development emphasis acknowledges that adolescence involves fundamental questions about who they are, what they value, and how they fit into the world. Group discussions naturally address these identity issues while providing diverse perspectives from peers facing similar developmental challenges.

Social justice awareness helps adolescents understand how societal factors such as discrimination, poverty, and educational inequity contribute to mental health challenges while building motivation for both personal change and social action.

Strength-based orientation counters the deficit-focused approaches often applied to teenagers with psychiatric conditions by identifying and building upon existing capabilities, interests, and positive relationships rather than focusing solely on problems and symptoms.

Creative Arts Therapy Adaptations

Adolescents often struggle with verbal expression of complex emotions, making creative arts approaches particularly valuable for this population. These interventions engage teenagers' natural creativity while providing alternative channels for communication and emotional processing.

Music therapy adaptations harness adolescents' strong connections to music for therapeutic purposes. Group members can share meaningful songs, write lyrics together, or use rhythm instruments to express emotions that feel too difficult to verbalize. Music provides common language that transcends cultural and socioeconomic differences.

Visual arts projects allow expression of internal experiences through drawing, painting, collage, or digital art creation. These activities work well for adolescents who feel self-conscious about verbal sharing while providing tangible products that can be revisited and discussed over time.

Drama and role-playing exercises help teenagers practice social skills, explore different perspectives, and work through challenging situations in safe environments. These activities appeal to adolescents' natural tendency toward experimentation and identity exploration.

Writing activities including journaling, poetry, and creative storytelling provide private reflection opportunities while building skills for emotional expression and self-awareness. Writing can be shared with the group or kept private, depending on individual comfort levels.

Movement and dance interventions address the embodied nature of adolescent experience while providing outlets for energy and physical expression. These activities can be particularly helpful for teenagers whose psychiatric conditions involve anxiety, depression, or trauma that affects their relationship with their bodies.

Case Example: Creative Arts for Adolescent Depression Group

Our adolescent depression group discovered that traditional talk therapy approaches felt too formal and adult-oriented for the six teenagers (ages 14-17) who were struggling with major depressive episodes. The group's transformation began when we introduced creative arts activities that allowed emotional expression through multiple modalities.

Ashley, a 16-year-old junior in high school, exemplified the challenges many teenagers face in verbalizing their emotional experiences. Her depression manifested through social withdrawal, academic decline, and persistent feelings of hopelessness that she described as "feeling empty inside" but couldn't elaborate further during traditional discussion formats.

Music sharing sessions became breakthrough moments for Ashley and other group members. Each session began with members sharing songs that reflected their current emotional states, leading to rich discussions about lyrics, musical styles, and personal connections to different artists. Ashley discovered that many of her peers connected with similar music themes about isolation, pain, and hope.

The group created **collaborative playlists** that represented their collective emotional journey, adding songs weekly that reflected both struggles and progress. This ongoing project provided continuity between sessions while creating shared cultural references that strengthened group bonds and communication.

Art therapy projects allowed Ashley to express her depression visually through drawings and collages that captured feelings she couldn't put into words. Her artwork progressed from dark, chaotic images early in treatment to more colorful, organized compositions that reflected her gradual mood improvement and increased hope.

Group **art exhibitions** displayed members' creative work (with permission) and provided opportunities for peer feedback and encouragement. These exhibitions celebrated creativity while normalizing emotional expression and building group pride in their collective artistic accomplishments.

Creative writing exercises helped Ashley develop vocabulary for her emotional experiences through poetry and short story writing. The group discovered that many members shared similar feelings and experiences, reducing isolation while building empathy and mutual understanding.

Ashley's transformation through creative arts engagement demonstrated the power of non-verbal therapeutic approaches for adolescents. Her depression scores improved significantly, her school attendance increased, and she developed friendships within the group that extended beyond formal treatment. Most importantly, she gained confidence in her ability to express and manage difficult emotions through multiple creative channels.

Social Skills Training Adaptations

Adolescent social skills training must account for the complex peer relationships, romantic interests, and family dynamics that characterize teenage social environments. Traditional adult-oriented social skills approaches often feel irrelevant to teenagers facing unique developmental challenges.

Peer interaction skills focus on the specific challenges of adolescent friendships including managing peer pressure, handling social conflicts, and navigating changing friendship dynamics. Group settings provide natural opportunities to practice these skills with age-matched peers.

Romantic relationship skills address the emerging interest in dating and intimate relationships that characterizes adolescence. These discussions must be age-appropriate while providing practical guidance about healthy relationship patterns and communication skills.

Family communication skills help teenagers navigate changing relationships with parents and siblings as they develop increased independence and autonomy. These skills often require balancing respectful communication with appropriate assertion of teenage needs and perspectives.

School-based social skills address the academic and social challenges of middle school and high school environments including interactions with teachers, group projects, and extracurricular activities that form major components of adolescent social experience.

Digital communication skills acknowledge the central role of social media, texting, and online interactions in teenage social life while addressing both opportunities and risks associated with digital communication.

Technology-Assisted Interventions

Modern adolescents are digital natives who feel more comfortable with technology-enhanced interventions than traditional paper-and-pencil approaches. Technology can support therapeutic goals while meeting teenagers where they naturally spend their time and energy.

Mental health apps designed specifically for adolescents provide mood tracking, coping skill reminders, and peer support features that extend group benefits between sessions. These apps must be carefully selected for age-appropriateness and evidence-based content.

Social media integration can support therapeutic goals through private group pages, shared resources, and peer support networks while maintaining appropriate boundaries and privacy protections. These platforms must be used carefully to avoid conflicts with confidentiality requirements.

Gaming elements including point systems, achievement badges, and collaborative challenges can motivate engagement with therapeutic activities while appealing to adolescents' competitive instincts and desire for recognition.

Virtual reality applications provide opportunities for exposure therapy, relaxation training, and social skills practice in controlled environments that feel engaging and modern to teenage participants.

Digital portfolios allow teenagers to document their therapeutic progress through photos, videos, and creative projects while building skills in self-reflection and goal tracking.

Case Example: Technology Integration for Social Anxiety

Our adolescent social anxiety group included five teenagers whose symptoms significantly interfered with school participation, peer relationships, and family functioning. Traditional exposure therapy approaches felt overwhelming to these anxious teens, requiring creative adaptations that used technology to bridge the gap between safe group settings and real-world social challenges.

Marcus, a 15-year-old sophomore, experienced severe social anxiety that prevented him from participating in class discussions, eating in the school cafeteria, or attending social events with peers. His avoidance behaviors had increased over the past year, limiting his academic and social development.

Virtual reality exposure allowed Marcus to practice social situations in controlled environments before attempting real-world interactions. He started with virtual presentations to small audiences, gradually building confidence before giving actual presentations in group settings and eventually in school classes.

The group used **social skills gaming** applications that provided structured practice opportunities for conversations, conflict resolution, and assertiveness skills. These games felt less threatening than role-playing exercises while providing immediate feedback and opportunities for repeated practice.

Peer support apps connected group members between sessions for encouragement and accountability. Marcus and his peers used secure messaging features to share successes, request support during challenging situations, and celebrate each other's progress toward social goals.

Progress tracking technology helped Marcus monitor his social anxiety levels, track exposure exercises, and document gradual improvements in his comfort levels across different social situations. This objective data provided motivation during difficult periods and evidence of progress when improvements felt slow.

Digital storytelling projects allowed Marcus to create videos documenting his journey with social anxiety while building skills in self-reflection and peer education. These projects gave him sense of purpose while reducing shame about his anxiety through helping others understand social anxiety challenges.

Marcus's successful integration of technology with traditional therapeutic approaches demonstrated how modern tools could support adolescent engagement with treatment. His social anxiety decreased significantly, his school participation improved, and he developed genuine friendships with other group members. The technology components provided bridges to real-world success rather than replacing human connection.

Case Example: Peer Support Groups for Eating Disorders

Our adolescent eating disorder support group required careful adaptation to address the competitive dynamics that can develop when teenagers with eating disorders share specific behaviors, weights, or food-related details. The group's success depended on creating supportive peer relationships while avoiding unhealthy comparisons or behavior escalation.

Emma, a 17-year-old with anorexia nervosa, initially used group sessions to compare her eating behaviors with other members and gain validation for her restrictive practices. Her competitive nature and perfectionism created risks for both her own recovery and negative influences on other group members.

Peer mentorship programs paired Emma with a slightly older young adult who had successfully recovered from an eating disorder. This mentorship provided hope and practical guidance while reducing competitive dynamics with current group members who were at similar stages of recovery.

The group developed **recovery-focused activities** that built positive peer relationships around healthy interests rather than eating disorder behaviors. These activities included creative projects, community service, and skill-building workshops that provided alternative sources of accomplishment and connection.

Strengths-based sharing replaced discussions about eating disorder behaviors with focus on personal strengths, interests, and recovery goals. Group members learned to support each other's positive qualities and achievements rather than bonding over symptoms or competitive behaviors.

Accountability partnerships helped group members support each other's recovery goals through regular check-ins, meal support, and encouragement during challenging situations. These partnerships provided practical assistance while building genuine friendships based on mutual care rather than eating disorder competition.

Family integration sessions helped group members practice communicating with parents about their needs and recovery goals while receiving peer support for family challenges. These sessions reduced isolation while building skills for healthy family relationships during recovery.

Emma's transformation from competitive eating disorder behaviors to supportive peer relationships demonstrated the power of carefully structured group interventions for adolescents with complex psychiatric conditions. Her recovery accelerated through peer support while her leadership in the group provided sense of purpose and meaning that supported long-term maintenance of healthy behaviors.

School Liaison and Transition Planning

Adolescent psychiatric treatment must coordinate closely with educational systems because school represents the primary developmental environment for teenagers. Effective group interventions include systematic approaches to school collaboration and transition planning.

Educational advocacy helps teenagers and families navigate special education services, 504 plans, and academic accommodations that support mental health recovery while maintaining educational progress. Group members can share experiences and strategies for working effectively with school personnel.

Teacher education provides school staff with information about psychiatric conditions and their impact on learning while building understanding and support for students receiving mental health treatment. This education reduces stigma while improving school-based support systems.

Peer support at school helps group members develop strategies for managing psychiatric symptoms in educational settings while building supportive peer relationships that extend beyond formal treatment programs.

Academic planning addresses how psychiatric conditions affect educational goals and career planning while maintaining hope and realistic expectations for academic achievement. These discussions help teenagers adapt their goals without abandoning their aspirations.

Transition preparation for post-secondary education, employment, or independent living must account for ongoing mental health needs while building confidence in teenagers' ability to manage their conditions successfully in adult settings.

Safety Protocols for Self-Harm Behaviors

Adolescent groups require specialized safety protocols because self-harm behaviors are common in this population and can be contagious within group settings. These protocols must balance safety with therapeutic benefit while maintaining group cohesion.

Risk assessment procedures identify teenagers at highest risk for self-harm while monitoring for changes in risk level throughout group participation. These assessments must be ongoing rather than one-time evaluations because adolescent risk factors can change rapidly.

Contagion prevention strategies reduce the likelihood that self-harm behaviors will spread among group members through detailed sharing or competitive dynamics. These strategies include clear guidelines about what information can be shared and how to discuss self-harm in therapeutic rather than triggering ways.

Crisis intervention plans outline specific steps for responding to self-harm disclosures or behaviors during group sessions while maintaining safety for all participants. These plans must be practiced and familiar to all staff members working with adolescent groups.

Family notification procedures clarify when and how parents or guardians will be contacted about safety concerns while balancing confidentiality with legal and ethical obligations to protect minor patients from harm.

Follow-up protocols ensure appropriate monitoring and support for group members who have engaged in self-harm behaviors while maintaining their connection to the group and ongoing treatment.

Family Involvement Strategies

Adolescent mental health treatment requires family involvement that balances teenagers' developing autonomy with parents' legitimate concerns and responsibilities. Group interventions must include systematic approaches to family engagement and support.

Family education sessions provide information about adolescent psychiatric conditions and their treatment while building understanding and support for teenagers' recovery efforts. These sessions help families understand normal adolescent development versus psychiatric symptoms.

Communication training helps families develop skills for discussing mental health topics without conflict while respecting teenagers' privacy and autonomy. These skills are essential for maintaining supportive family relationships during treatment.

Boundary setting assists families in establishing appropriate limits and expectations while allowing teenagers increasing independence and responsibility for their mental health management.

Crisis planning involves families in developing plans for managing psychiatric emergencies while clarifying roles and responsibilities for parents, teenagers, and treatment providers.

Long-term planning helps families prepare for ongoing mental health management as teenagers transition to adulthood and assume greater responsibility for their own care.

Developmental Considerations

Successful adolescent group interventions must account for the unique developmental tasks and challenges that characterize this life stage while adapting therapeutic approaches accordingly.

Identity formation represents the central developmental task of adolescence, requiring group interventions that support healthy identity development while addressing psychiatric symptoms that can interfere with this process.

Cognitive development continues throughout adolescence, with implications for abstract thinking, risk assessment, and decision-making abilities that affect both psychiatric symptoms and treatment engagement.

Peer relationships become increasingly important during adolescence, making group interventions particularly powerful while also requiring careful attention to peer dynamics and social pressures.

Family relationships change significantly during adolescence as teenagers develop increasing autonomy, requiring treatment approaches that support both individual development and family adaptation to these changes.

Future orientation develops during adolescence, making goal-setting and future planning important components of group interventions while accounting for the uncertainty and anxiety that often accompany thinking about the future.

Building Resilience

Adolescent psychiatric groups provide unique opportunities for building resilience factors that support long-term mental health and successful transition to adulthood.

Coping skills development teaches practical strategies for managing stress, difficult emotions, and challenging situations while building confidence in teenagers' ability to handle future challenges independently.

Support network building helps teenagers develop and maintain relationships that support their mental health and recovery goals while providing resources for ongoing support after formal treatment ends.

Problem-solving skills prepare teenagers for the increasing independence and responsibility that characterize young adulthood while building confidence in their ability to navigate complex challenges.

Self-advocacy skills teach teenagers how to communicate their needs effectively and seek appropriate help when needed while building confidence in their ability to manage their mental health as adults.

Hope and meaning development addresses existential questions that often arise during adolescence while building sense of purpose and motivation for continued growth and recovery.

Pathways to Success

Adolescent psychiatric group interventions represent investments in the future—both for individual teenagers and for the communities they will eventually serve as adults. Your role in facilitating these groups carries special significance because effective intervention during these formative years can alter life trajectories in profound and lasting ways.

The energy, creativity, and resilience that teenagers bring to group settings create opportunities for rapid change and growth that may not be available at other life stages. Your nursing knowledge and skills provide foundation for maximizing these opportunities while ensuring safety and therapeutic benefit for all group participants.

Clinical Applications

- Integrated theoretical models combining interpersonal and feminist perspectives address both relational development and power dynamics affecting adolescent mental health
- Creative arts adaptations provide alternative channels for emotional expression that appeal to teenagers' natural creativity and address verbal communication difficulties
- Technology-assisted interventions meet adolescents where they naturally engage while supporting therapeutic goals through modern, appealing formats
- School liaison and transition planning ensure continuity between treatment and educational settings while building long-term success strategies

- Safety protocols for self-harm behaviors balance risk management with therapeutic benefit while preventing contagion within group settings
- Family involvement strategies support both adolescent autonomy and appropriate parental engagement in treatment and recovery planning

Chapter 10: Geriatric Mental Health Groups

The intersection of aging and mental health creates unique challenges that require specialized group interventions adapted for older adults' cognitive abilities, sensory limitations, and life experiences. Geriatric mental health groups address not only psychiatric symptoms but also the complex losses, transitions, and medical comorbidities that characterize later life, requiring you to integrate knowledge of aging processes with psychiatric nursing expertise.

Your nursing background provides essential advantages in geriatric mental health groups because you understand how medical conditions affect cognitive function, how medications interact to influence mood and behavior, and how physical limitations impact participation in therapeutic activities. You also recognize that depression and anxiety in older adults often masquerade as cognitive impairment or medical complaints, requiring careful assessment and intervention approaches.

Evidence Base for Geriatric Group Therapy

Research consistently demonstrates that group therapy approaches can be highly effective for older adults, often showing outcomes equal to or better than individual therapy while providing additional benefits of social connection and peer support that address the isolation commonly experienced by older adults (23). Studies reveal particular effectiveness for depression, anxiety, and grief-related conditions that frequently affect this population.

Depression treatment studies show that group cognitive-behavioral therapy and interpersonal therapy produce significant improvements in older adults with major depressive disorder, with effect sizes comparable to antidepressant medications but with lower side effect profiles and greater acceptability among patients who prefer psychosocial interventions.

Anxiety intervention research indicates that group approaches can effectively address generalized anxiety, panic disorder, and specific phobias in older adults while providing exposure opportunities that feel safer and more supportive than individual treatment approaches.

Cognitive stimulation evidence demonstrates that structured group activities can slow cognitive decline and improve quality of life for individuals with mild cognitive impairment and early dementia while providing respite and support for family caregivers.

Social engagement benefits extend beyond symptom improvement to include reduced healthcare utilization, decreased nursing home placement, and improved overall functioning that supports aging in place and maintains independence longer.

Cost-effectiveness analyses show that group interventions for older adults provide significant economic benefits through reduced medical costs, decreased emergency department visits, and delayed institutional placement while improving quality of life and functional status.

Reminiscence Therapy Protocols

Reminiscence therapy harnesses older adults' rich life experiences and intact long-term memories to promote emotional well-being, social connection, and sense of meaning while addressing depression and isolation that can accompany aging (24). These structured approaches validate lifetime experiences while building current coping resources.

Life review processes guide systematic exploration of personal history, major life events, and important relationships while identifying themes of resilience, accomplishment, and meaning that can support current emotional well-being and coping efforts.

Structured reminiscence activities use prompts such as historical events, music from different decades, or photographs to stimulate memory sharing while ensuring all group members have opportunities to participate regardless of their specific life experiences or backgrounds.

Intergenerational sharing connects older adults with younger volunteers or family members to share life stories and wisdom while building mutual understanding and appreciation across age groups.

Legacy projects help older adults document their life stories, family histories, or important lessons learned while creating meaningful products that can be shared with family members or preserved for future generations.

Themed reminiscence sessions focus on specific topics such as work experiences, family traditions, or historical events while providing structure that guides sharing and ensures relevance for all group members.

Case Example: Reminiscence Therapy for Late-Life Depression

Our geriatric depression group included eight community-dwelling older adults (ages 72-89) whose depression symptoms had developed following significant losses including spouse death, health problems, and retirement transitions. Traditional therapy approaches felt foreign to this generation that valued stoicism and self-reliance over emotional expression.

Margaret, an 84-year-old retired librarian, exemplified the presentation common among older adults with depression—she minimized her emotional distress while attributing her symptoms to "normal aging" and expressing skepticism about mental health treatment. Her depression had worsened following her husband's death two years earlier, leading to social withdrawal and functional decline.

Structured life review sessions provided framework for Margaret to share her 60-year marriage, career achievements, and parenting experiences while identifying patterns of resilience and coping that had sustained her through previous challenges. These sessions reframed her current struggles within the context of her lifetime strengths and resources.

The group discovered through **historical reminiscence** that Margaret and other members had lived through the Great Depression, World War II, and significant social changes that required tremendous adaptability and strength. These shared experiences created bonds while highlighting their proven capacity for surviving difficult circumstances.

Family tradition sharing helped Margaret reconnect with meaningful activities and relationships that had been neglected since her husband's death. She rediscovered her love of cooking family recipes and began hosting holiday gatherings that provided purpose and social connection.

Legacy project work involved Margaret creating a cookbook of family recipes with accompanying stories about their origins and significance. This project honored her husband's memory while providing meaningful activity that connected her with family members and preserved important traditions.

Music-based reminiscence using songs from Margaret's young adult years triggered positive memories and emotions while providing group bonding experiences around shared cultural references. These sessions often ended with singing together, creating joyful experiences that countered depressive mood states.

Margaret's transformation through reminiscence therapy demonstrated the power of strength-based approaches for older adults. Her depression scores improved significantly, her social engagement increased, and she developed new friendships within the group that continued after formal treatment ended. Most importantly, she reconnected with her sense of identity and purpose beyond her role as a grieving widow.

Cognitive Stimulation Activities

Cognitive stimulation groups provide structured mental exercises and social engagement that can slow cognitive decline while improving quality of life for older adults with mild cognitive impairment or early dementia (25). These activities must be challenging enough to provide benefit while remaining achievable for participants with varying cognitive abilities.

Memory exercises including word games, story completion, and photo recognition activities stimulate cognitive function while providing enjoyable group experiences that build confidence and social connection.

Problem-solving activities such as puzzles, brain teasers, and logic games provide mental stimulation while encouraging collaborative problem-solving that builds social bonds and mutual support among group members.

Creative activities including art projects, music participation, and creative writing engage multiple cognitive domains while providing opportunities for self-expression and accomplishment that boost self-esteem and mood.

Current events discussions stimulate cognitive engagement while maintaining connections to contemporary world events and community happenings that support continued learning and intellectual curiosity.

Skill-building workshops teaching new abilities such as computer use, crafts, or hobbies provide cognitive challenges while building sense of accomplishment and purpose that supports overall well-being and life satisfaction.

Grief and Loss Support Groups

Older adults experience multiple losses including deaths of spouses, friends, and family members, as well as losses of independence, roles, and physical abilities that require specialized grief support approaches adapted for this population's unique needs and experiences.

Complicated grief interventions address prolonged or intense grief reactions that interfere with functioning while providing support for working through grief processes that may feel overwhelming or insurmountable.

Multiple loss support acknowledges that older adults often face several losses simultaneously or in close succession, requiring approaches that address cumulative grief and the compound impact of multiple significant losses.

Anticipatory grief work helps older adults prepare for expected losses such as declining health or terminal diagnoses while maintaining hope and meaning during difficult transitions.

Disenfranchised grief recognition validates losses that may not be socially recognized such as pet deaths, loss of independence, or changes in cognitive function that represent significant losses requiring grief work and support.

Meaning-making processes help older adults find purpose and significance in their loss experiences while building connections between their grief and their broader life stories and spiritual beliefs.

Case Example: Grief Support Following Spouse Loss

Our widowhood support group included six older adults (ages 68-85) who had lost spouses within the past two years and were struggling with depression, anxiety, and adjustment difficulties that interfered with their ability to rebuild meaningful lives as single individuals.

Robert, a 78-year-old retired engineer, had been married for 52 years when his wife died suddenly from a heart attack. His grief was complicated by guilt about not recognizing her symptoms earlier and by complete unfamiliarity with household tasks she had managed throughout their marriage.

Grief education sessions helped Robert understand that his intense emotional responses, physical symptoms, and cognitive difficulties represented normal grief reactions rather than signs of mental illness or personal weakness. This education reduced his fear about his grief while building hope for eventual healing.

The group provided **peer support** from others who understood the unique challenges of late-life widowhood including loneliness, practical difficulties, and social changes that occur when couples lose their social networks after spouse death.

Practical skill building addressed Robert's need to learn household management, cooking, and social planning skills that had been his wife's responsibilities. Group members shared knowledge and resources while providing encouragement for learning new skills at an advanced age.

Memorial activities helped Robert find meaningful ways to honor his wife's memory while continuing his own life. He created a scholarship fund in her name and volunteered at organizations she had supported, providing ongoing connection to her while building new purpose and meaning.

Social reconstruction work addressed Robert's need to develop new social connections and activities as a single person after decades of couple-focused social life. The group provided initial social network while helping members develop confidence for broader community engagement.

Robert's grief work demonstrated the unique challenges and opportunities of late-life loss. While his grief was profound and long-lasting, his eventual adjustment included new friendships, expanded social skills, and deeper appreciation for life that enriched his remaining years. The group support was essential for navigating this difficult transition.

Case Example: Anxiety Management in Late Life

Our geriatric anxiety group addressed the specific presentations and treatment needs of eight older adults whose anxiety symptoms often differed significantly from younger populations' presentations. Many group members had developed anxiety late in life following health problems, losses, or life transitions rather than experiencing lifelong anxiety conditions.

Dorothy, an 82-year-old former teacher, developed severe anxiety following a fall that resulted in hip fracture and temporary nursing home placement. Her anxiety focused on fears of falling again, losing independence, and becoming a burden to her family, leading to avoidance behaviors that limited her activities and social engagement.

Anxiety education helped Dorothy understand how trauma from her fall had triggered anxiety responses and how avoidance behaviors were maintaining and worsening her fears. This education reduced her shame about feeling anxious while building understanding of anxiety as treatable medical condition.

Gradual exposure exercises adapted for older adults' physical limitations helped Dorothy gradually resume activities she had been avoiding since her fall. The group provided support and encouragement for taking appropriate risks while maintaining safety precautions.

Relaxation training including progressive muscle relaxation, deep breathing, and guided imagery provided practical skills for managing anxiety symptoms while accommodating physical limitations such as arthritis that made some traditional relaxation techniques difficult.

Cognitive restructuring addressed catastrophic thinking patterns about aging, health, and independence while building more balanced perspectives on risk and safety that allowed continued engagement in meaningful activities.

Safety planning helped Dorothy develop realistic strategies for preventing falls while maintaining active lifestyle. This planning reduced anxiety by providing concrete steps for risk reduction while avoiding excessive restrictions that would limit quality of life.

Dorothy's anxiety improvement demonstrated the importance of addressing both emotional and practical aspects of late-life anxiety. Her group participation provided peer support while building skills for managing anxiety that supported her continued independence and engagement in community activities.

Social Engagement Programs

Isolation and loneliness represent significant risk factors for depression and cognitive decline in older adults, making social engagement a central component of geriatric mental health interventions that extends beyond symptom reduction to include community building and support network development.

Community integration activities help older adults maintain connections to their communities while building new relationships and interests that provide meaning and purpose during later life transitions.

Intergenerational programs connect older adults with younger community members through mentoring, tutoring, or shared activities that provide mutual benefits while reducing age segregation and building understanding across generations.

Volunteer opportunities harness older adults' skills and experience while providing sense of purpose and contribution that supports self-esteem and life satisfaction during retirement years.

Interest-based groups organize around shared hobbies, activities, or learning goals while providing social connection based on common interests rather than shared problems or deficits.

Mutual support networks help group members develop ongoing relationships that provide practical assistance and emotional support beyond formal treatment periods while building community resilience and social capital.

Environmental Modifications

Successful geriatric mental health groups require environmental adaptations that accommodate sensory impairments, mobility limitations, and cognitive changes that can affect older adults' ability to participate effectively in group activities.

Lighting considerations ensure adequate illumination for reading and visual activities while reducing glare that can be problematic for older adults with vision changes or cataracts.

Seating arrangements provide comfortable, supportive chairs arranged in circles that promote interaction while accommodating mobility aids such as walkers or wheelchairs.

Acoustic modifications reduce background noise and improve sound quality through microphone systems or room treatments that help older adults with hearing impairments participate effectively in group discussions.

Timing adaptations schedule groups during times when older adults feel most alert and energetic while allowing adequate time for transportation and preparation.

Material modifications use large print, high contrast colors, and simple formats that accommodate vision changes and cognitive limitations while maintaining dignity and age-appropriateness.

Collaboration with Long-Term Care

Geriatric mental health groups often need to coordinate with long-term care facilities, home health services, and family caregivers to ensure continuity of care and support for group members' ongoing mental health needs.

Facility-based groups adapt interventions for nursing home or assisted living settings while addressing the unique challenges and opportunities of institutional environments.

Caregiver education provides family members and professional caregivers with information about mental health conditions and interventions while building support for continued therapeutic engagement.

Transition planning addresses moves between different levels of care while maintaining therapeutic relationships and continuing mental health interventions across settings.

Quality of life focus emphasizes functional improvement and life satisfaction rather than cure-oriented goals that may be unrealistic for older adults with chronic conditions or progressive illnesses.

Palliative approaches integrate mental health interventions with end-of-life care while addressing spiritual and existential concerns that become prominent during final life stages.

Medical Integration

Geriatric mental health groups must account for the complex medical conditions and medication regimens that characterize this population while coordinating with primary care providers and specialists to ensure comprehensive care.

Medication review identifies drugs that may contribute to depression or anxiety while working with prescribers to optimize regimens that support both physical and mental health.

Chronic disease management addresses how conditions such as diabetes, heart disease, or chronic pain affect mental health while building coping strategies that support overall health and quality of life.

Cognitive assessment distinguishes between depression-related cognitive changes and dementia while adapting interventions appropriately for each individual's cognitive abilities and limitations.

Physical activity integration incorporates appropriate exercise and movement into mental health interventions while accommodating physical limitations and safety concerns.

Preventive care coordination ensures that group members maintain appropriate medical screening and preventive care while addressing mental health symptoms that might interfere with self-care.

Cultural Considerations for Older Adults

Geriatric mental health groups must account for the unique cultural backgrounds and historical experiences of older adults while respecting generational differences in attitudes toward mental health treatment and help-seeking behaviors.

Generational attitudes acknowledge that many older adults were raised during times when mental health stigma was greater and treatment options were limited, requiring approaches that respect these perspectives while providing current information.

Cultural diversity addresses the varying ethnic, religious, and socioeconomic backgrounds of older adults while ensuring that interventions are culturally appropriate and respectful of different traditions and values.

Communication styles adapt to generational preferences for formal communication and respect for authority while building therapeutic relationships that honor older adults' wisdom and experience.

Family involvement navigates complex family dynamics and varying cultural expectations about family roles in healthcare decisions while respecting older adults' autonomy and dignity.

Spiritual considerations acknowledge the increased importance of spirituality and religion for many older adults while incorporating these resources into mental health interventions when appropriate and desired.

Wisdom Through Experience

Geriatric mental health groups offer unique opportunities to witness the resilience, wisdom, and continued capacity for growth that characterize many older adults despite their mental health challenges. Your role in facilitating these groups provides privileged access to life stories and perspectives that can inform both professional practice and personal understanding of aging processes.

The richness of older adults' life experiences and their proven capacity for surviving multiple challenges creates powerful therapeutic resources that distinguish geriatric groups from other populations. Your nursing expertise in managing complex medical and psychosocial needs provides foundation for maximizing these resources while ensuring safe and effective interventions.

Essential Implementation Elements

- Evidence-based geriatric group therapy shows effectiveness equal to individual treatment while providing additional social connection benefits that address isolation common in older adults
- Reminiscence therapy protocols harness intact long-term memories and rich life experiences to promote healing while building current coping resources and sense of meaning
- Cognitive stimulation activities provide structured mental exercises that slow decline while improving quality of life for individuals with mild cognitive impairment or early dementia
- Grief and loss support groups address multiple simultaneous losses common in later life while providing peer support from others facing similar challenges
- Environmental modifications accommodate sensory impairments and mobility limitations while maintaining dignity and promoting effective participation
- Medical integration addresses complex health conditions and medication effects that influence mental health presentation and treatment response in older adults

Chapter 11: Dual Diagnosis Group Interventions

The co-occurrence of mental health and substance use disorders presents complex treatment challenges that require specialized group interventions addressing both conditions simultaneously rather than treating them as separate problems. Dual diagnosis groups recognize that psychiatric symptoms and substance use often maintain each other in cycles that cannot be broken without integrated approaches that address the underlying connections between mental health and addiction.

Your nursing background provides essential advantages in dual diagnosis treatment because you understand how substances interact with psychiatric medications, how withdrawal symptoms can mimic or worsen psychiatric conditions, and how medical complications of substance use affect overall health and treatment engagement. You also recognize that many individuals use substances as self-medication for untreated psychiatric symptoms, requiring approaches that address both the underlying mental health needs and the substance use behaviors.

Integrated Treatment Approaches

Effective dual diagnosis treatment requires integration of mental health and substance abuse interventions rather than parallel or sequential treatment of separate conditions (26). Research consistently demonstrates that integrated approaches produce better outcomes than traditional sequential models that require individuals to achieve sobriety before addressing psychiatric conditions.

Simultaneous treatment addresses both conditions concurrently through interventions that recognize their interconnected nature while building skills for managing both psychiatric symptoms and substance use triggers within unified treatment frameworks.

Motivational approaches acknowledge that individuals with dual diagnosis often have different levels of motivation for addressing mental health versus substance use issues, requiring interventions that meet people where they are while building motivation for change in both areas.

Harm reduction principles recognize that complete abstinence may not be immediately achievable for all individuals while supporting any positive changes that reduce risk and improve functioning, building momentum toward more significant recovery goals.

Trauma-informed care addresses the high prevalence of trauma among individuals with dual diagnosis while ensuring that treatment approaches do not retraumatize participants through confrontational or punitive interventions.

Stage-wise interventions adapt treatment intensity and focus based on individuals' readiness for change while providing appropriate support for different stages of recovery from both mental health and substance use perspectives.

Triggers and Coping Skills Worksheets

Understanding the relationship between triggers and substance use provides foundation for developing effective coping strategies that address both immediate crisis situations and long-term recovery maintenance. Group settings allow peer sharing of trigger identification and coping strategy development.

Internal trigger identification helps group members recognize emotional states, physical sensations, and thought patterns that increase their risk for substance use while building awareness of early warning signs that require intervention.

External trigger mapping identifies environmental factors, social situations, and contextual cues that increase substance use risk while developing strategies for avoiding or managing these situations safely.

Coping skills hierarchy organizes coping strategies from immediate crisis interventions to long-term lifestyle changes while providing multiple options for different situations and individual preferences.

Skill practice sessions provide opportunities to rehearse coping strategies in group settings while receiving feedback and support from peers who understand similar challenges and situations.

Effectiveness tracking monitors which coping strategies work best for individual group members while identifying patterns and preferences that guide ongoing skill development and refinement.

Case Example: Integrated Treatment for Depression and Alcohol Use Disorder

Our dual diagnosis group included eight individuals with co-occurring depression and substance use disorders who had experienced multiple treatment failures using traditional sequential approaches that required sobriety before addressing mental health symptoms.

Michael, a 42-year-old construction worker, exemplified the challenges of dual diagnosis treatment. His depression had begun in his twenties following job loss and relationship problems, leading to increasing alcohol use as self-medication for depressive symptoms. Previous treatment attempts had failed because he couldn't maintain sobriety long enough for antidepressant medications to work effectively.

Integrated assessment revealed that Michael's drinking patterns closely followed his depression cycles—increased alcohol use during depressive episodes followed by shame and increased depression about his drinking, creating self-perpetuating cycles that traditional treatment approaches had not addressed.

Motivation building helped Michael understand that his depression and alcohol use were connected problems requiring simultaneous attention rather than viewing sobriety as prerequisite for mental health treatment. This reframing reduced his shame while building hope that integrated treatment could be more effective.

Coping skills development focused on alternatives to alcohol for managing depressive symptoms including behavioral activation, social support utilization, and crisis intervention strategies that could be used during high-risk situations.

Medication coordination involved careful timing of antidepressant treatment with alcohol reduction rather than requiring complete sobriety before starting psychiatric medications. This approach provided hope and symptom relief that supported motivation for continued alcohol reduction.

Peer support from other group members who understood the challenges of managing both conditions provided validation and practical strategies that individual therapy could not offer. Michael learned from others' experiences while contributing his own insights to group members facing similar challenges.

Michael's recovery through integrated treatment demonstrated the power of addressing dual diagnosis conditions simultaneously. His depression improved significantly while his alcohol use decreased from daily drinking to occasional lapses that no longer derailed his overall recovery progress. The group support was essential for maintaining motivation during the gradual improvement process.

Relapse Prevention Planning

Dual diagnosis relapse prevention requires planning for both psychiatric symptom recurrence and substance use episodes while recognizing that relapse in one area often triggers problems in the other domain.

Early warning sign identification teaches group members to recognize subtle changes in mood, thinking, or behavior that may indicate increased risk for both psychiatric symptoms and substance use before full relapse occurs.

Trigger management strategies provide specific techniques for managing high-risk situations while building confidence in group members' ability to navigate challenging circumstances without returning to previous levels of dysfunction.

Support system activation helps group members identify and utilize appropriate resources during crisis situations while building networks that understand both mental health and substance use challenges.

Emergency planning provides step-by-step instructions for managing psychiatric emergencies and substance use crises while maintaining safety and minimizing damage to long-term recovery goals.

Recovery maintenance activities establish ongoing practices that support both mental health stability and substance use recovery while providing structure and meaning that reduce risk for both types of relapse.

Recovery Support Groups

Peer support represents a crucial component of dual diagnosis treatment because individuals with similar experiences can provide understanding, encouragement, and practical guidance that professional treatment alone cannot offer.

Shared experience validation reduces isolation and shame while building understanding that dual diagnosis conditions are common and treatable rather than representing personal failures or moral weaknesses.

Practical strategy sharing allows group members to learn from each other's successes and failures while building repertoires of coping strategies and recovery techniques that have been tested by peers facing similar challenges.

Accountability partnerships provide ongoing support and motivation between formal treatment sessions while creating relationships that support long-term recovery maintenance and crisis intervention.

Celebration and recognition of recovery milestones and achievements builds group culture that values progress while providing positive reinforcement for continued recovery efforts.

Mentorship opportunities allow individuals with longer recovery to support newer group members while providing sense of purpose and meaning that supports their own recovery maintenance.

Case Example: Relapse Prevention for Bipolar Disorder and Cocaine Use

Our dual diagnosis group for individuals with bipolar disorder and stimulant use disorders addressed the complex interactions between mood episodes and substance use while building skills for managing both conditions during high-risk periods.

Sandra, a 35-year-old marketing professional, had experienced multiple hospitalizations for manic episodes that were often precipitated or worsened by cocaine use during hypomanic periods. Her pattern involved using cocaine to enhance the energy and productivity of early hypomania, leading to full manic episodes that required hospitalization and created significant life disruption.

Pattern identification helped Sandra recognize the early signs of mood elevation that increased her risk for cocaine use while building understanding of how stimulant use could trigger manic episodes that undid months of stability.

Alternative strategies for managing hypomanic energy included increased exercise, creative projects, and social activities that provided stimulation and excitement without the risks associated with cocaine use.

Medication adherence planning addressed Sandra's tendency to stop taking mood stabilizers during hypomanic periods when she felt "too good" to need medication, recognizing that this pattern increased both mood episode risk and cocaine use vulnerability.

Support system education helped Sandra's family and friends recognize early warning signs of both mood changes and increased substance use risk while learning how to provide appropriate support without enabling or creating conflict.

Crisis intervention planning provided specific steps for managing high-risk situations including immediate interventions for cocaine cravings during mood episodes and emergency procedures for managing manic symptoms that could lead to dangerous substance use.

Sandra's development of effective relapse prevention skills demonstrated the importance of addressing the interaction between psychiatric symptoms and substance use rather than treating them as separate problems. Her understanding of how mood changes affected her cocaine vulnerability allowed her to implement early interventions that prevented full relapses in both areas.

Case Example: Trauma-Informed Approach for PTSD and Alcohol Use

Our trauma-focused dual diagnosis group addressed the high prevalence of trauma among individuals with co-occurring substance use disorders while ensuring that treatment approaches supported healing rather than retraumatization.

David, a 29-year-old military veteran, developed PTSD following combat exposure and began using alcohol to manage nightmares, hypervigilance, and intrusive memories. His drinking had escalated to daily use that interfered with work and relationships while providing only temporary relief from trauma symptoms.

Trauma education helped David understand how alcohol temporarily reduced PTSD symptoms while ultimately worsening them through interference with natural recovery processes and creation of additional life problems that increased stress and trauma responses.

Safety planning addressed both psychological safety during trauma processing and physical safety during alcohol withdrawal while building David's confidence in his ability to manage trauma symptoms without substances.

Grounding techniques provided alternatives to alcohol for managing dissociation, flashbacks, and overwhelming emotions while building skills that could be used in any situation without legal or health consequences.

Exposure therapy adaptations for dual diagnosis included careful coordination of trauma processing with alcohol reduction while ensuring that neither intervention overwhelmed David's coping capacity or triggered relapse in either area.

Peer support from other veterans with similar experiences provided validation and practical strategies while reducing isolation and building connections based on shared military experience and understanding of combat trauma.

David's recovery through trauma-informed dual diagnosis treatment demonstrated the importance of addressing underlying trauma that drove his substance use rather than focusing only on drinking behaviors. His PTSD symptoms improved significantly while his alcohol use decreased to occasional social drinking that no longer interfered with his functioning.

Motivational Interviewing Techniques

Motivational interviewing provides evidence-based approach for addressing ambivalence about change that is common among individuals with dual diagnosis conditions while supporting autonomous decision-making and building intrinsic motivation for recovery.

Exploring ambivalence acknowledges that individuals often have mixed feelings about giving up substances or addressing mental health symptoms while helping them explore both sides of their ambivalence without pressure or judgment.

Rolling with resistance avoids confrontational approaches that often increase defensiveness while supporting individuals' autonomy and right to make their own decisions about treatment and recovery goals.

Building motivation focuses on individuals' own reasons for change rather than external pressure while supporting their values and goals that may be inconsistent with continued substance use or untreated mental health symptoms.

Change planning helps individuals develop specific, achievable goals while building confidence in their ability to make positive changes in both mental health and substance use areas.

Supporting self-efficacy builds individuals' confidence in their ability to achieve their goals while providing realistic feedback about progress and challenges that maintains hope without creating unrealistic expectations.

Medication-Assisted Treatment Education

Many individuals with dual diagnosis benefit from medications that address both psychiatric symptoms and substance use disorders, requiring education about these treatments while addressing concerns and misconceptions that might interfere with treatment engagement.

Addiction medication education covers treatments such as methadone, buprenorphine, and naltrexone while addressing stigma and misconceptions about medication-assisted treatment that might prevent individuals from accessing these effective interventions.

Psychiatric medication integration addresses how addiction medications interact with psychiatric treatments while coordinating care between addiction medicine and psychiatric providers to ensure safe and effective treatment.

Side effect management prepares individuals for potential side effects of both addiction and psychiatric medications while providing strategies for managing these effects without discontinuing beneficial treatments.

Monitoring requirements explains blood tests, clinic visits, and other monitoring needs associated with medication-assisted treatment while building understanding of these requirements as safety measures rather than punitive restrictions.

Long-term planning addresses questions about duration of medication-assisted treatment while building realistic expectations about recovery timelines and ongoing medication needs.

Trauma-Informed Approaches

The high prevalence of trauma among individuals with dual diagnosis requires treatment approaches that recognize trauma's impact while avoiding retraumatization through inappropriate interventions or environmental factors.

Universal trauma screening identifies trauma histories among all group members while providing appropriate referrals and safety planning for individuals with significant trauma backgrounds.

Safety emphasis ensures that group environments feel physically and emotionally safe while building trust and predictability that supports trauma recovery alongside addiction and mental health treatment.

Choice and control provides individuals with options about their participation level and treatment approaches while respecting their autonomy and avoiding power struggles that can trigger trauma responses.

Collaboration involves individuals as partners in their treatment planning while respecting their expertise about their own experiences and needs rather than imposing external treatment goals or approaches.

Cultural responsiveness addresses how trauma intersects with cultural identity while ensuring that treatment approaches respect diverse backgrounds and experiences rather than imposing dominant cultural assumptions.

Family and Social System Interventions

Dual diagnosis conditions affect entire family and social systems while requiring interventions that address these broader impacts and build support for recovery efforts.

Family education provides information about dual diagnosis conditions while building understanding and reducing blame that often develops when families don't understand the relationship between mental health and substance use.

Communication training helps families develop skills for providing support without enabling while learning how to set appropriate boundaries that protect their own well-being.

Crisis planning involves families in developing responses to psychiatric emergencies and substance use crises while clarifying roles and responsibilities during high-risk situations.

Recovery support teaches families how to recognize and reinforce progress while avoiding inadvertent sabotage of recovery efforts through well-meaning but counterproductive behaviors.

Self-care education addresses the stress and burden that families experience while providing resources and support for their own mental health and well-being.

Building Integrated Recovery

Dual diagnosis recovery requires integration of mental health and substance use treatment approaches while building lifestyle changes that support both types of recovery simultaneously. Your nursing expertise provides foundation for understanding these complex interactions while supporting individuals through the challenging process of addressing multiple conditions.

The group setting provides peer support and shared learning opportunities that individual treatment cannot replicate while building community connections that support long-term recovery maintenance and prevent isolation that increases risk for both psychiatric symptoms and substance use relapse.

Clinical Integration Points

- Integrated treatment approaches address mental health and substance use disorders simultaneously rather than treating them as separate sequential problems
- Triggers and coping skills development recognizes interconnected nature of psychiatric symptoms and substance use while building unified recovery strategies
- Relapse prevention planning addresses both psychiatric symptom recurrence and substance use episodes while recognizing their interactive effects
- Motivational interviewing techniques support autonomous decision-making while building intrinsic motivation for change in both mental health and substance use areas
- Medication-assisted treatment education addresses stigma while coordinating addiction medications with psychiatric treatments for comprehensive care
- Trauma-informed approaches recognize high trauma prevalence while ensuring that treatment supports healing rather than retraumatization

Chapter 12: Cultural Competency in Group Practice

The increasing diversity of mental health service recipients requires psychiatric nurses to develop sophisticated understanding of how cultural factors influence group participation, therapeutic relationships, and treatment outcomes. Cultural competency goes beyond surface-level awareness of different ethnic groups to include deep appreciation for how cultural identity shapes individuals' understanding of mental illness, appropriate help-seeking behaviors, and acceptable treatment approaches.

Your nursing education provides foundation for cultural competency through emphasis on holistic care and respect for individual differences, but group practice requires additional skills for managing cultural dynamics among multiple participants while ensuring that interventions remain culturally appropriate and effective for diverse populations (27).

Cultural Competency Framework

Effective cultural competency requires systematic approach that moves beyond cultural awareness to include cultural knowledge, cultural skills, and cultural encounters that build genuine understanding and respect for diverse populations and their mental health needs.

Cultural awareness involves recognition of your own cultural background, biases, and assumptions while understanding how these factors influence your perceptions of patients and therapeutic relationships. This self-awareness provides foundation for recognizing when cultural differences may be affecting group dynamics or treatment effectiveness.

Cultural knowledge includes specific information about different cultural groups' beliefs about mental illness, traditional healing practices, family structures, and communication styles that influence how individuals experience and respond to psychiatric symptoms and treatment approaches.

Cultural skills encompass practical abilities for conducting culturally sensitive assessments, adapting interventions for different populations, and communicating effectively across cultural differences while building therapeutic relationships that respect diverse worldviews and values.

Cultural encounters involve direct interaction with individuals from different cultural backgrounds while seeking opportunities to learn from these experiences and build understanding that goes beyond textbook knowledge to include real-world appreciation for cultural diversity.

Cultural desire represents genuine motivation to become culturally competent while recognizing that this process requires ongoing commitment to learning and growth rather than one-time training or superficial multicultural awareness.

Cultural Assessment Tools

Systematic cultural assessment provides foundation for adapting group interventions to meet diverse participants' needs while identifying potential barriers to treatment engagement and developing strategies for culturally appropriate care.

ETHNIC framework guides cultural assessment through Explanation (patient's understanding of illness), Treatment (previous treatments tried), Healers (traditional healers consulted), Negotiate (treatment preferences), Intervene (cultural adaptations needed), and Collaborate (involving cultural supports).

Cultural genogram mapping explores family cultural background, immigration history, acculturation levels, and cultural conflicts that may influence mental health symptoms and treatment engagement while identifying cultural resources and supports available to group members.

Language assessment evaluates English proficiency, preferred communication language, and need for interpreter services while understanding how language barriers might affect group participation and therapeutic relationships.

Religious and spiritual assessment explores religious affiliation, spiritual practices, and beliefs about mental illness and healing that may influence treatment acceptability while identifying spiritual resources that can support recovery efforts.

Acculturation evaluation assesses level of adaptation to dominant culture while understanding how acculturation stress may contribute to mental health symptoms and affect treatment preferences and engagement.

Case Example: Culturally Adapted Depression Group for Latina Women

Our depression support group for Latina women required significant cultural adaptations to address the specific beliefs, values, and experiences that influenced how these women understood and sought help for their mental health symptoms.

Carmen, a 45-year-old immigrant from El Salvador, exemplified the cultural factors that affected treatment engagement. She understood her depression symptoms as "nervios" (nerves) rather than mental illness and felt shame about seeking help outside her family for what she viewed as personal weakness rather than medical condition.

Cultural reframing of depression helped Carmen understand that "nervios" represented valid medical condition that required treatment rather than personal failing that should be managed through willpower or religious faith alone. This reframing reduced shame while building acceptance of treatment approaches.

Family involvement respected Carmen's cultural values about collective decision-making while building support for her treatment participation. Group sessions included family education components that helped relatives understand depression and support Carmen's recovery efforts.

Religious integration acknowledged Carmen's Catholic faith while incorporating prayer, spiritual reflection, and discussion of how faith could support rather than conflict with mental health treatment. This integration reduced perceived conflicts between religious beliefs and psychological interventions.

Gender-specific focus addressed the unique stressors that Latina women face including domestic responsibilities, childcare burdens, immigration stress, and financial concerns while building culturally appropriate coping strategies and support networks.

Language accommodation provided group sessions in Spanish while using culturally relevant metaphors and concepts that resonated with group members' cultural backgrounds and life experiences rather than relying on direct translations of English-language interventions.

Carmen's response to culturally adapted treatment demonstrated the importance of respecting cultural beliefs while providing effective mental health interventions. Her depression improved significantly while her cultural identity remained intact and strengthened through the treatment process.

Language and Communication Adaptations

Effective cross-cultural group practice requires sophisticated understanding of how language differences affect therapeutic relationships and group dynamics while developing strategies for ensuring effective communication across diverse populations.

Interpreter utilization involves working effectively with professional interpreters while understanding how interpretation affects group dynamics, confidentiality, and therapeutic relationships among group members who speak different languages.

Nonverbal communication awareness recognizes that eye contact, personal space, touch, and other nonverbal behaviors have different meanings across cultures while adapting facilitation style to respect diverse communication preferences and norms.

Indirect communication styles acknowledge that many cultures value indirect communication over direct confrontation while adapting group interventions to accommodate these preferences without losing therapeutic effectiveness.

Silence interpretation understands that silence may have different meanings across cultures including respect, reflection, disagreement, or confusion while responding appropriately to these varied meanings rather than assuming lack of engagement.

Metaphor and storytelling utilize culturally relevant imagery and narratives that resonate with different cultural backgrounds while making therapeutic concepts accessible and meaningful across diverse populations.

Incorporating Cultural Healers

Many cultural groups maintain traditional healing practices that can complement psychiatric treatment while providing familiar and acceptable approaches to mental health that may be more culturally congruent than Western therapeutic interventions alone.

Traditional healer collaboration involves respectful partnership with curanderos, medicine people, religious leaders, and other cultural healers while coordinating care to ensure that traditional and Western approaches support rather than conflict with each other.

Healing practice integration incorporates traditional ceremonies, herbal remedies, energy healing, and other cultural practices into group interventions while maintaining safety and therapeutic effectiveness.

Spiritual healing recognition acknowledges the role of spiritual practices in mental health recovery while respecting diverse religious traditions and beliefs about the relationship between spirituality and psychological well-being.

Cultural ceremony adaptation modifies traditional healing practices for group settings while maintaining their cultural integrity and therapeutic value for participants who find meaning and healing through these approaches.

Elder involvement includes respected community elders in group activities while honoring their wisdom and cultural knowledge as resources for healing and guidance that complement professional mental health expertise.

Case Example: Integration of Traditional Healing for Native American Veterans

Our PTSD treatment group for Native American veterans required integration of traditional healing practices with evidence-based trauma treatment while respecting tribal sovereignty and cultural protocols that govern mental health healing in Native communities.

Joseph, a 34-year-old Army veteran from the Lakota tribe, had experienced combat trauma during multiple deployments but found that traditional PTSD treatments felt disconnected from his cultural identity and understanding of spiritual balance and community healing.

Traditional healing integration involved collaboration with tribal healers who provided cleansing ceremonies, talking circles, and spiritual guidance that complemented cognitive-behavioral trauma therapy while addressing Joseph's understanding of trauma as spiritual as well as psychological injury.

Community healing approaches recognized that individual trauma affects entire tribal communities while incorporating family and community members into healing processes that honored Lakota values about collective responsibility and support.

Cultural trauma acknowledgment addressed how historical trauma from colonization, forced assimilation, and cultural suppression contributed to Joseph's vulnerability to combat PTSD while building understanding of intergenerational trauma transmission and healing.

Sacred space creation ensured that group meetings honored Native protocols for creating sacred healing space while incorporating smudging, prayer, and other spiritual practices that supported therapeutic work within culturally appropriate contexts.

Warrior tradition honoring respected Joseph's identity as a warrior within Lakota tradition while addressing how this identity could support rather than conflict with trauma healing and mental health recovery.

Joseph's healing through integrated traditional and Western approaches demonstrated the power of culturally responsive treatment that honored both professional expertise and cultural wisdom in addressing complex trauma presentations.

Case Example: Islamic Cultural Adaptations for Anxiety Treatment

Our anxiety management group for Muslim community members required adaptations that respected Islamic beliefs and practices while providing effective treatment for anxiety disorders that interfered with religious observance and daily functioning.

Fatima, a 28-year-old graduate student wearing hijab, experienced severe social anxiety that interfered with her academic performance and religious community participation. Her anxiety was complicated by concerns about whether mental health treatment conflicted with Islamic teachings about trusting in Allah and accepting divine will.

Religious integration explored how Islamic teachings about trust in Allah could coexist with taking appropriate action to address medical conditions while framing mental health treatment as fulfilling religious obligations to care for the body and mind that Allah has entrusted to each individual.

Prayer schedule accommodation ensured that group meeting times did not conflict with daily prayers while incorporating Islamic concepts of mindfulness and reflection that aligned with anxiety management techniques.

Cultural modesty respect honored Islamic guidelines about gender interaction and physical modesty while adapting relaxation and mindfulness exercises to remain culturally appropriate and comfortable for observant Muslim participants.

Family involvement navigated cultural expectations about family involvement in healthcare decisions while respecting both individual autonomy and collective family values that characterize many Muslim communities.

Halal considerations ensured that any recommended supplements or medications met Islamic dietary requirements while addressing concerns about substance use that might conflict with religious prohibitions.

Fatima's improvement through culturally adapted anxiety treatment demonstrated how mental health interventions could support rather than conflict with religious observance while providing effective symptom relief that enhanced her ability to participate fully in both academic and religious communities.

Religious and Spiritual Considerations

Spirituality and religious faith represent important resources for many individuals' mental health recovery while requiring careful integration that respects diverse beliefs without imposing particular religious perspectives on group participants.

Spiritual assessment explores individuals' religious background, current spiritual practices, and beliefs about the relationship between spirituality and mental health while identifying spiritual resources that can support recovery efforts.

Faith-based coping recognizes prayer, meditation, scripture reading, and other spiritual practices as legitimate coping strategies while building understanding of how these practices can complement professional mental health treatment.

Religious conflict resolution addresses situations where religious beliefs appear to conflict with mental health treatment while helping individuals find ways to honor both their faith and their mental health needs.

Interfaith dialogue manages groups that include members from different religious traditions while fostering respect and understanding across diverse spiritual perspectives and practices.

Secular adaptation ensures that individuals who do not identify with religious traditions feel equally respected and included while adapting spiritual concepts into secular frameworks that provide similar benefits without religious content.

Interpreter Use in Groups

Working with interpreters in group settings presents unique challenges that require specialized skills and protocols to ensure effective communication while maintaining group dynamics and therapeutic effectiveness.

Interpreter selection involves choosing interpreters with mental health experience while ensuring cultural and linguistic competency that goes beyond basic language translation to include understanding of cultural concepts and therapeutic processes.

Pre-session preparation includes briefing interpreters about group goals, therapeutic concepts, and cultural sensitivities while establishing protocols for handling confidential information and maintaining professional boundaries.

Seating arrangements position interpreters to facilitate communication while minimizing disruption to group dynamics and ensuring that both verbal and nonverbal communication can be effectively interpreted.

Group dynamic management addresses how interpretation affects group flow and member interaction while developing strategies for maintaining group cohesion and therapeutic focus despite language barriers.

Confidentiality protocols ensure that interpreters understand and maintain confidentiality requirements while addressing potential conflicts when interpreters have community connections with group members.

LGBTQIA+ Cultural Competency

Sexual and gender minority populations face unique challenges in group settings that require specialized understanding and interventions to ensure safe and effective treatment while addressing minority stress and identity-related concerns.

Identity affirmation creates group environments where diverse sexual orientations and gender identities are respected and validated while addressing internalized stigma and minority stress that contribute to mental health symptoms.

Coming out support provides appropriate resources for individuals exploring or disclosing their sexual orientation or gender identity while respecting individual choices about disclosure and identity expression.

Family rejection issues addresses the high rates of family rejection experienced by LGBTQIA+ individuals while building alternative support networks and coping strategies for managing family conflict and loss.

Discrimination trauma recognizes how experiences of discrimination, harassment, and violence affect mental health while building resilience and coping strategies for managing ongoing minority stress.

Transition support provides appropriate resources for transgender individuals while ensuring that group environments are supportive and affirming of diverse gender expressions and transition experiences.

Socioeconomic Cultural Factors

Economic status represents a cultural factor that significantly affects mental health symptoms and treatment engagement while requiring adaptations that address practical barriers and different life experiences across socioeconomic groups.

Resource accessibility addresses how poverty affects ability to attend groups, access medications, and engage in therapeutic activities while developing strategies for overcoming financial barriers to treatment.

Work schedule accommodation recognizes that many individuals work multiple jobs or irregular schedules that interfere with traditional group meeting times while developing flexible scheduling that supports treatment engagement.

Transportation barriers addresses lack of reliable transportation that prevents group attendance while developing solutions such as public transportation resources, ride-sharing arrangements, or location modifications.

Childcare needs acknowledges that many individuals cannot attend groups without childcare while developing solutions that support parents' treatment engagement without creating additional financial burden.

Insurance limitations navigates restrictions on mental health coverage while advocating for appropriate services and developing strategies for continuing care despite financial constraints.

Building Cultural Bridges

Successful cultural competency in group practice requires ongoing commitment to learning and growth while building authentic relationships with diverse communities and populations that extend beyond formal treatment settings.

Community engagement involves participating in cultural events, community organizations, and educational opportunities that build understanding and relationships with diverse populations outside of clinical settings.

Cultural mentorship seeks guidance from individuals with lived experience in different cultures while building relationships that provide ongoing learning and consultation about culturally appropriate care.

Continuing education pursues formal training in cultural competency while staying current with research and best practices for working with diverse populations in mental health settings.

Self-reflection maintains ongoing awareness of personal biases and cultural assumptions while seeking feedback about cultural competency from colleagues, supervisors, and community members.

Advocacy involvement supports policies and practices that improve mental health care access and quality for diverse populations while addressing systemic barriers that prevent equitable treatment.

Reflections on Diversity

Cultural competency in group practice represents both professional obligation and personal growth opportunity that enriches your understanding of human diversity while improving your effectiveness as a psychiatric nurse. The willingness to step outside your cultural comfort zone and learn from individuals whose experiences differ significantly from your own creates opportunities for profound personal and professional development.

The group setting provides unique laboratory for observing how cultural differences can enrich therapeutic experiences while learning to navigate the complexities of multicultural group dynamics. Your role as facilitator requires balancing respect for cultural diversity with maintenance of therapeutic focus and group cohesion.

Cultural Practice Foundations

- Cultural competency framework requires systematic development of awareness, knowledge, skills, encounters, and desire rather than superficial multicultural training

- Cultural assessment tools provide structured approaches for understanding how cultural factors influence mental health symptoms and treatment preferences
- Language and communication adaptations ensure effective therapeutic relationships while respecting diverse communication styles and preferences
- Traditional healer integration respects cultural healing practices while coordinating care to support rather than conflict with psychiatric treatment
- Religious and spiritual considerations honor diverse faith traditions while identifying spiritual resources that support mental health recovery
- Interpreter use in groups requires specialized protocols that maintain therapeutic effectiveness while ensuring accurate cross-cultural communication

Chapter 13: Group Facilitation Skills for Nurses

The art of group facilitation demands a unique blend of clinical knowledge, interpersonal sensitivity, and practical management skills that transform ordinary meetings into healing experiences. As a psychiatric nurse leading therapeutic groups, you orchestrate complex human dynamics while maintaining focus on treatment goals, managing time constraints, and responding to the unexpected crises that inevitably arise when people gather to share their most vulnerable experiences.

Your nursing background provides distinct advantages in group facilitation because you understand how medical conditions affect behavior, how medications influence group participation, and how to recognize when individual needs require immediate attention that might disrupt group processes. You also possess the clinical judgment necessary to balance competing demands while maintaining therapeutic safety for all participants.

Leadership Styles in Group Therapy

Effective group leadership requires flexibility to adapt your style based on group developmental stage, member characteristics, and therapeutic objectives while maintaining consistent therapeutic presence that builds trust and promotes healing (28). Research identifies several leadership approaches that can be effective depending on specific group needs and circumstances.

Democratic leadership involves shared decision-making and collaborative goal-setting that respects group members' autonomy while providing structure and guidance necessary for therapeutic progress. This approach works particularly well with motivated adults who benefit from increased responsibility for their recovery processes.

Authoritative leadership provides clear structure and direction while maintaining warmth and support that helps anxious or confused group members feel safe and contained. This style often works best during group formation stages or with populations that benefit from external structure and guidance.

Laissez-faire leadership offers minimal direction while allowing groups to develop their own processes and solutions to problems. This hands-off approach can be effective with highly motivated, experienced group members but may feel overwhelming for individuals with severe symptoms or limited group experience.

Transformational leadership inspires group members to exceed their perceived limitations while building hope and motivation for change that extends beyond symptom management to include personal growth and meaning-making.

Situational leadership adapts style based on immediate group needs and circumstances while maintaining therapeutic focus and safety. This flexible approach requires sophisticated assessment skills and clinical judgment to match leadership responses to group requirements.

Opening and Closing Rituals

Structured beginnings and endings create therapeutic containers that distinguish group time from everyday experiences while building group identity and promoting psychological safety necessary for therapeutic work.

Opening rituals establish group focus and prepare members for therapeutic engagement through consistent activities that signal transition from external concerns to internal reflection and group connection. These rituals might include moment of silence, check-in rounds, mindfulness exercises, or affirmations that help members shift attention to therapeutic goals.

Check-in procedures provide opportunities for members to share current emotional states, significant events since the last session, and goals for the current meeting while helping facilitators assess individual needs and group readiness for planned activities.

Transition activities help members move from individual preoccupations to group focus through exercises that build connection and shared attention. These might include partner sharing, group movement, or creative activities that engage multiple senses and promote present-moment awareness.

Closing rituals provide opportunities to process session content, consolidate learning, and transition back to daily life while maintaining connections forged during group time. Effective closings include reflection on session highlights, commitment to between-session activities, and appreciation for group members' courage and contributions.

Continuity building connects current sessions to previous meetings and future goals while helping members track their progress and maintain motivation for continued group participation and therapeutic work.

Case Example: Opening Rituals for Trauma Recovery Group

Our trauma recovery group required carefully designed opening rituals that created safety and predictability for eight women whose histories of abuse and violence had left them hypervigilant and easily triggered by unexpected changes or intense emotions.

Patricia, a 34-year-old survivor of domestic violence, exemplified the need for structured beginnings that helped group members transition from the outside world to therapeutic focus while managing anxiety about sharing vulnerable experiences with others.

The **grounding ritual** began each session with a five-minute mindfulness exercise that helped members connect with their bodies and present-moment experience rather than remaining caught in trauma memories or anticipatory anxiety about group participation.

Safety affirmations reminded group members of their right to control their participation level, leave the room if needed, and request support during difficult moments. These affirmations reduced anxiety while building confidence in members' ability to maintain safety during emotional discussions.

Intention setting invited each member to identify what they hoped to gain from the session while providing opportunities to request specific support or indicate need for gentle participation due to difficult weeks or triggering events.

The **connection circle** involved members sharing one word that described their current emotional state while making eye contact with each other, building bonds and mutual awareness that supported group cohesion and empathy.

Resource reminder reviewed coping skills and support options available during and after sessions while reinforcing members' capacity to manage difficult emotions that might arise during group discussions.

Patricia's response to structured openings demonstrated the power of predictable rituals for trauma survivors. The consistent format reduced her anxiety while building trust in group safety that allowed her to gradually share more vulnerable experiences and accept support from other members.

Managing Dominant Members

Every group includes individuals who tend to monopolize discussion time, offer excessive advice, or dominate through physical presence, humor, or emotional intensity that can interfere with other members' participation and therapeutic progress.

Early intervention addresses dominant behaviors before they become entrenched patterns by gently redirecting excessive participation while validating the member's contributions and maintaining therapeutic relationships.

Time structuring provides clear guidelines about sharing time and discussion limits while ensuring equitable participation opportunities for all group members regardless of their communication styles or comfort levels.

Role clarification helps dominant members understand their impact on others while building awareness of how their behavior affects group dynamics and other members' therapeutic experiences.

Positive channeling redirects dominant tendencies toward constructive roles such as peer mentoring, group leadership assistance, or modeling appropriate self-disclosure that benefits rather than hinders group processes.

Individual consultation addresses persistent dominant behaviors through private conversations that explore underlying needs driving excessive participation while developing strategies for more balanced group engagement.

Encouraging Quiet Participants

Silent or minimally participating group members may feel overwhelmed, anxious, depressed, or culturally conditioned to defer to others, requiring specific interventions that respect their participation style while encouraging gradual engagement.

Gentle invitations provide opportunities for quiet members to participate without pressure while respecting their right to observe and learn through listening rather than verbal sharing.

Alternative participation offers non-verbal ways to contribute through writing exercises, art activities, or small group discussions that feel less threatening than large group verbal sharing.

Strength identification recognizes and verbally acknowledges quiet members' contributions such as attentive listening, emotional support through presence, or insights shared during less formal moments.

Cultural sensitivity considers whether silence reflects cultural communication patterns, language barriers, or respect for authority rather than lack of engagement or resistance to treatment.

Gradual engagement builds participation slowly through increasingly comfortable sharing opportunities while celebrating small steps and avoiding pressure that might increase anxiety or withdrawal.

Case Example: Balancing Participation in Depression Group

Our depression support group included twelve members with varying communication styles and comfort levels, requiring careful balance between ensuring adequate sharing time while managing dominant personalities and encouraging quiet participants.

Marcus dominated discussions through lengthy stories and frequent advice-giving that prevented others from sharing, while Susan rarely spoke despite obvious emotional responses to group content and clear investment in other members' progress.

Structured sharing rounds provided equal time allocations for each member while preventing Marcus from monopolizing discussion through his tendency to elaborate extensively on every topic introduced.

The talking stone method involved passing an object that designated speaking turns while creating natural pauses and transitions that gave quieter members opportunities to contribute without competing for floor time.

Marcus received **individual feedback** about his impact on group dynamics while exploring how his advice-giving might reflect his own need for control and purpose during his depression recovery.

Small group activities paired Susan with one or two other members for sharing exercises that felt less overwhelming than addressing the entire group while building confidence for larger group participation.

Written reflections provided alternative ways for Susan to share insights through journal entries read aloud, anonymous submissions, or written responses to group questions that honored her preference for thoughtful, prepared communication.

The **appreciation ritual** at session endings specifically acknowledged both verbal and non-verbal contributions while helping all members recognize how their presence and attention supported others' healing processes.

Both Marcus and Susan developed more balanced participation patterns through these interventions—Marcus learned to share more concisely while asking questions that drew out other members, and Susan gradually increased her verbal contributions while maintaining her valuable role as empathetic listener and emotional support provider.

Case Example: Managing Emotional Intensity in Anxiety Group

Our generalized anxiety group regularly experienced moments of high emotional intensity when members shared panic attacks, phobic reactions, or overwhelming worry episodes that could trigger similar responses in other anxious participants.

During one session, Jennifer's description of a severe panic attack triggered visible anxiety responses in three other group members, threatening to escalate into group-wide panic that could undermine therapeutic safety and progress.

Immediate grounding involved guiding the entire group through breathing exercises and grounding techniques that interrupted the anxiety spiral while maintaining group cohesion and safety.

Emotional regulation teaching provided practical tools for managing intense emotions during group sessions while building skills that members could use in daily life when experiencing overwhelming anxiety.

Containment strategies helped Jennifer process her panic experience without overwhelming detail that might trigger others while validating her courage in sharing difficult experiences with the group.

Group support mobilization encouraged members to offer appropriate support and encouragement while avoiding advice-giving or minimizing that could increase rather than reduce anxiety levels.

Processing opportunities addressed the group's collective response to Jennifer's panic episode while building understanding of anxiety contagion and developing strategies for supporting each other without becoming overwhelmed.

The group learned to **surf emotional waves** together rather than being overwhelmed by individual members' intense experiences while building skills for managing anxiety both individually and collectively.

Handling Emotional Intensity

Groups provide powerful catalysts for emotional expression that can feel overwhelming for both individuals experiencing intense emotions and other group members witnessing these expressions.

Emotional safety protocols establish guidelines for managing intense emotions while maintaining group stability and ensuring that emotional expression serves therapeutic rather than retraumatizing purposes.

Containment techniques help individuals express emotions safely while preventing emotional flooding that overwhelms coping capacity and interferes with therapeutic processing and integration.

Group support activation mobilizes other members' empathy and encouragement while teaching appropriate ways to provide emotional support that helps rather than overwhelms distressed individuals.

Professional intervention recognizes when individual crisis needs require immediate attention that temporarily shifts group focus while maintaining safety and therapeutic benefit for all participants.

Integration processing helps groups learn from emotional intensity experiences while building collective capacity for supporting each other through difficult emotions and challenging therapeutic material.

Co-Facilitation Models

Working with co-facilitators provides multiple perspectives and skills while offering backup support during challenging group situations and modeling healthy professional relationships for group members.

Complementary skills partnerships combine facilitators with different strengths such as process expertise paired with content knowledge, or medical background combined with psychotherapy training that enhances overall group leadership capacity.

Gender balance considerations provide both male and female perspectives that can be particularly beneficial for groups addressing relationship issues, trauma recovery, or gender-specific mental health concerns.

Cultural diversity in facilitation teams demonstrates respect for diverse backgrounds while providing multiple cultural perspectives that enhance cultural competency and group accessibility.

Training partnerships pair experienced facilitators with those developing group leadership skills while providing mentorship opportunities and ensuring continuity of care during transition periods.

Communication protocols establish clear agreements about facilitation roles, intervention strategies, and decision-making processes while preventing confusion or conflict that could undermine group stability and therapeutic effectiveness.

Supervision and Consultation

Group facilitation generates complex ethical, clinical, and interpersonal challenges that require ongoing supervision and consultation to ensure safe and effective practice while supporting facilitator development and preventing burnout.

Regular supervision provides opportunities to process challenging group situations, explore countertransference reactions, and develop intervention strategies while ensuring adherence to professional standards and ethical guidelines.

Peer consultation offers perspectives from colleagues with group experience while building professional support networks that reduce isolation and provide diverse viewpoints on difficult clinical situations.

Crisis consultation ensures access to immediate guidance during group emergencies while establishing protocols for managing safety concerns, ethical dilemmas, and complex clinical presentations that exceed individual expertise.

Continuing education maintains current knowledge about group therapy research and techniques while building specialized skills for working with specific populations or addressing particular clinical challenges.

Self-care planning addresses the emotional demands of group work while developing strategies for maintaining personal well-being and professional effectiveness over time.

Time Management Strategies

Effective group facilitation requires sophisticated time management that balances planned activities with spontaneous therapeutic opportunities while ensuring adequate attention to all group members and therapeutic objectives.

Session structure planning allocates time for opening rituals, main activities, processing discussions, and closing procedures while maintaining flexibility for unexpected therapeutic moments or crisis interventions.

Activity pacing adjusts timing based on group energy, engagement levels, and therapeutic needs while avoiding rushed transitions or prolonged activities that lose focus or overwhelm participants.

Individual attention balance ensures adequate time for each member's needs while preventing sessions from being dominated by single individuals or issues that don't benefit the entire group.

Process versus content decisions involve moment-to-moment choices about focusing on planned activities versus emerging group dynamics that may offer superior therapeutic opportunities.

Transition management provides smooth movement between activities while maintaining therapeutic momentum and group engagement throughout session duration.

Building Therapeutic Relationships

The foundation of effective group facilitation rests on authentic therapeutic relationships that balance professional boundaries with genuine human connection while modeling healthy relationship patterns for group members.

Genuine presence involves showing up authentically while maintaining appropriate professional boundaries that provide safety and structure necessary for therapeutic work.

Empathetic attunement requires accurate perception of individual and group emotional states while responding appropriately to support therapeutic progress and emotional safety.

Boundary maintenance protects both facilitators and group members through clear guidelines about appropriate relationships, self-disclosure, and contact outside group settings.

Cultural responsiveness adapts facilitation style to honor diverse communication preferences and cultural norms while maintaining therapeutic effectiveness across different populations.

Professional growth involves ongoing development of facilitation skills while seeking feedback and supervision that supports excellence in group leadership and patient care.

Technology Integration

Modern group facilitation increasingly involves technology components that can enhance therapeutic experiences while requiring new skills for managing virtual interactions and hybrid group formats.

Virtual group platforms provide access to individuals who cannot attend in-person sessions while requiring adaptations for building therapeutic relationships and managing group dynamics through digital interfaces.

Hybrid group formats combine in-person and virtual participants while addressing technical challenges and ensuring equitable participation opportunities regardless of attendance format.

Digital therapeutic tools supplement group activities through apps, online resources, and interactive technologies while maintaining focus on human connection and therapeutic relationships.

Privacy and security considerations ensure confidentiality and safety in digital environments while complying with healthcare regulations and protecting sensitive mental health information.

Technical troubleshooting requires basic skills for managing common technology problems while having backup plans for continuing therapeutic work when technical difficulties arise.

Practical Applications

Group facilitation represents both art and science that develops through practice, supervision, and commitment to ongoing learning about human dynamics and therapeutic interventions. Your nursing expertise provides excellent foundation for this work while requiring additional skills specific to group processes and leadership.

The rewards of effective group facilitation include witnessing profound healing experiences while building professional skills that enhance your effectiveness across all nursing practice areas. The challenge involves managing complex human dynamics while maintaining therapeutic focus and safety for all participants.

Foundational Skills

- Leadership styles require flexibility to adapt approaches based on group developmental stages and member characteristics while maintaining consistent therapeutic presence
- Opening and closing rituals create therapeutic containers that distinguish group time from everyday experiences while building safety and group identity
- Managing dominant members requires early intervention and positive channeling while encouraging quiet participants through gentle invitations and alternative participation methods
- Emotional intensity management involves safety protocols and containment techniques while mobilizing group support and professional intervention when needed
- Co-facilitation models provide complementary skills and perspectives while requiring clear communication protocols and shared decision-making agreements
- Supervision and consultation ensure safe practice and professional development while addressing complex ethical and clinical challenges inherent in group work

Chapter 14: Safety and Crisis Management in Groups

The therapeutic intensity of group settings creates unique safety challenges that require specialized assessment skills, intervention protocols, and crisis management strategies adapted for multiple participants experiencing varying levels of distress simultaneously. Group crises can escalate rapidly through emotional contagion while involving complex interpersonal dynamics that demand immediate, skilled responses to protect all participants while maintaining therapeutic benefits.

Your nursing background provides essential advantages in group crisis management because you understand medical emergencies, medication effects that might contribute to crisis situations, and systematic approaches to risk assessment and intervention that can be adapted for group settings where individual crises affect multiple people simultaneously.

Environmental Safety Protocols

Creating physically and emotionally safe group environments requires systematic attention to environmental factors that influence both crisis prevention and crisis management while ensuring that safety measures support rather than hinder therapeutic processes (29).

Physical environment assessment evaluates room layout, furniture placement, exit accessibility, and potential safety hazards while ensuring that group spaces feel welcoming and therapeutic rather than institutional or threatening.

Emergency equipment access ensures availability of first aid supplies, emergency communication devices, and crisis intervention resources while maintaining discrete placement that doesn't create anxiety or institutional atmosphere.

Privacy protection balances confidentiality needs with safety requirements while ensuring that crisis interventions can be implemented without compromising other group members' therapeutic experiences or confidentiality.

Lighting and acoustics create calming environments that reduce anxiety and agitation while ensuring adequate visibility and sound quality for effective communication during both routine sessions and crisis situations.

Accessibility considerations accommodate individuals with disabilities while ensuring that all group members can participate safely and comfortably regardless of physical limitations or mobility needs.

Risk Assessment Procedures

Systematic risk assessment provides foundation for crisis prevention while identifying individuals who may require additional support or modified interventions to participate safely in group settings.

Suicide risk evaluation uses standardized assessment tools and clinical interview techniques to identify individuals at risk for self-harm while developing appropriate safety planning and intervention strategies.

Violence risk assessment evaluates potential for aggressive or threatening behavior toward other group members or facilitators while implementing appropriate precautions and intervention protocols.

Substance use screening identifies individuals whose alcohol or drug use might impair judgment or create safety concerns during group participation while addressing these issues through appropriate referrals and safety planning.

Mental status evaluation assesses cognitive functioning, reality testing, and emotional stability while identifying individuals whose psychiatric symptoms might interfere with safe group participation or crisis management.

Medical condition review considers how physical health problems, medications, or medical treatments might affect group participation or crisis presentations while coordinating with healthcare providers as appropriate.

Case Example: Managing Suicidal Crisis in Depression Group

Our depression support group faced a crisis situation when Robert, a 52-year-old group member, disclosed active suicidal ideation with specific plans during a routine check-in, requiring immediate intervention while maintaining group safety and therapeutic benefit for other participants.

Robert's **crisis disclosure** occurred during opening check-in when he stated that he had been "thinking about ending it all" and had researched methods online, triggering immediate safety concerns that required balancing his individual needs with group stability.

Immediate safety assessment involved private consultation with Robert while arranging coverage for group continuation, determining imminent risk level, and developing appropriate intervention strategies that protected his safety while minimizing disruption to other group members.

Group communication provided appropriate information to remaining members about Robert's safety status while maintaining confidentiality and helping them process their own reactions to his crisis disclosure without overwhelming them with details.

Crisis intervention included safety planning, emergency contact notification, and coordination with mental health crisis services while ensuring that Robert felt supported rather than punished for his honest disclosure of suicidal thoughts.

Follow-up planning addressed Robert's return to group participation while ensuring appropriate ongoing safety monitoring and support that maintained his connection to group resources during his recovery from acute suicidal crisis.

The **group processing** in subsequent sessions helped members understand crisis response procedures while building confidence in group safety and their ability to support each other during difficult periods without becoming overwhelmed by others' crises.

Robert's crisis management demonstrated the importance of having clear protocols while maintaining therapeutic relationships and group cohesion during emergency situations that could otherwise traumatize or overwhelm other group participants.

De-escalation Scripts

Structured verbal interventions can effectively reduce tension and prevent crisis escalation while maintaining therapeutic relationships and group safety during challenging situations that might otherwise require more restrictive interventions.

Validation scripts acknowledge individuals' emotional experiences while redirecting attention toward problem-solving and coping strategies rather than allowing continued escalation of distressing emotions.

Redirection techniques guide conversations away from triggering topics or interactions while maintaining respect for individuals' autonomy and avoiding power struggles that might increase agitation.

Grounding prompts help individuals reconnect with present-moment reality while reducing anxiety, panic, or dissociation that might be contributing to crisis presentations.

Collaboration language engages individuals as partners in crisis resolution while avoiding authoritarian approaches that might increase resistance or defensive responses.

Safety reminders reinforce group norms and safety protocols while helping individuals recall their coping resources and support options during moments of overwhelming distress.

Safety Planning Worksheets

Written safety plans provide concrete resources for managing crisis situations while involving individuals in developing personalized strategies that build confidence and self-efficacy for crisis management.

Warning sign identification helps individuals recognize early symptoms of crisis development while building awareness that can support early intervention and prevention of full crisis episodes.

Coping strategy lists identify specific techniques that have been effective for individual crisis management while providing easy reference during times when thinking clearly becomes difficult due to emotional overwhelm.

Support person contacts compile names and phone numbers of individuals who can provide assistance during crises while ensuring that support resources are readily available when professional help is not immediately accessible.

Professional resource information includes crisis hotlines, emergency services, and mental health providers while ensuring that individuals know how to access appropriate help during different types of emergencies.

Environmental safety modifications address specific risk factors in individuals' living situations while developing strategies for creating safer environments that reduce crisis risk and support recovery.

Case Example: De-escalation for Bipolar Group Crisis

Our bipolar disorder support group experienced escalating conflict between two members that threatened group safety and required immediate de-escalation to prevent verbal aggression from escalating to physical confrontation or emotional trauma for other participants.

The **conflict trigger** occurred when James criticized Maria's medication compliance decisions, leading to defensive responses that escalated into personal attacks and angry accusations that activated both individuals' bipolar symptoms and triggered anxiety in other group members.

Immediate intervention involved physical positioning between the conflicted members while using calm, low voice tones and non-threatening body language to reduce tension and prevent further escalation of aggressive behaviors.

Validation statements acknowledged both members' frustration while redirecting their attention away from personal attacks toward underlying concerns about medication decisions and treatment approaches that had triggered the conflict.

Grounding techniques helped both individuals reconnect with present-moment reality while reducing emotional intensity that was interfering with rational communication and problem-solving abilities.

Group involvement engaged other members in supporting de-escalation through modeling calm behavior and offering perspectives that helped conflicted members recognize common ground rather than focusing on their differences.

Resolution planning involved both members in developing agreements about future communication while building understanding of how their bipolar symptoms might affect their interactions during group sessions.

The **learning opportunity** processing helped all group members understand conflict de-escalation techniques while building confidence in their ability to manage interpersonal difficulties without requiring external intervention or group disruption.

Case Example: Medical Emergency Response

Our anxiety disorders group faced a medical emergency when Sandra experienced what appeared to be a heart attack during a panic attack discussion, requiring immediate medical response while managing other members' anxiety reactions and maintaining group safety.

Sandra's **symptom presentation** included chest pain, shortness of breath, dizziness, and numbness that could indicate either severe panic attack or cardiac emergency, requiring immediate assessment and appropriate medical response while avoiding assumptions about psychiatric versus medical causation.

Emergency protocols included calling emergency medical services while monitoring Sandra's vital signs and providing emotional support that reduced her panic while ensuring that potential cardiac symptoms received appropriate medical evaluation.

Group management involved helping other anxious members understand the situation while preventing panic contagion that could overwhelm multiple participants and interfere with emergency response efforts.

Family notification contacted Sandra's emergency contact while coordinating with medical personnel and providing relevant information about her psychiatric history and current medications that might affect emergency treatment decisions.

Session continuation addressed remaining members' anxiety about Sandra's condition while processing their own fears about medical emergencies and panic attacks that the situation had triggered for several participants.

Follow-up planning included communication with Sandra about her medical evaluation results while coordinating her return to group participation and addressing any ongoing anxiety about medical emergencies that might affect her treatment progress.

The emergency response demonstrated the importance of maintaining medical assessment skills while leading psychiatric groups and having clear protocols for managing situations that blur the boundaries between psychiatric and medical emergencies.

Emergency Response Protocols

Systematic emergency procedures ensure appropriate responses to various crisis situations while maintaining clarity about roles, responsibilities, and communication requirements during high-stress situations that can impair decision-making.

Communication procedures establish clear protocols for contacting emergency services, notifying supervisors, and informing family members while ensuring that confidentiality requirements are balanced with safety needs and legal obligations.

Documentation requirements specify information that must be recorded during and after emergency situations while ensuring that legal and regulatory requirements are met without interfering with immediate crisis response needs.

Staff role clarification designates specific responsibilities for different team members during emergencies while ensuring that all necessary tasks are covered and avoiding confusion that might compromise emergency response effectiveness.

Follow-up procedures address post-crisis activities including incident debriefing, ongoing safety monitoring, and treatment plan modifications while ensuring continuity of care and prevention of future crisis situations.

Training requirements ensure that all staff members have appropriate emergency response skills while maintaining current certifications and competencies necessary for safe group practice.

Post-Crisis Debriefing

Systematic processing of crisis events provides learning opportunities while addressing the emotional impact on all involved parties and identifying system improvements that can prevent similar situations or improve future crisis responses.

Individual debriefing addresses the emotional impact on the individual who experienced crisis while identifying factors that contributed to the situation and developing strategies for future crisis prevention and management.

Group processing helps other members understand crisis events while addressing their emotional reactions and building confidence in group safety and crisis management procedures.

Staff debriefing reviews emergency response effectiveness while identifying system improvements and addressing staff emotional reactions to crisis situations that might affect future performance or well-being.

System evaluation examines organizational factors that might have contributed to crisis development while implementing policy or procedure changes that could prevent similar situations or improve crisis response effectiveness.

Learning integration incorporates crisis experience into ongoing training and education while building organizational capacity for effective crisis management and prevention.

Legal and Ethical Considerations

Crisis management in group settings involves complex legal and ethical issues that require understanding of professional obligations, regulatory requirements, and ethical principles that guide appropriate decision-making during emergency situations.

Confidentiality limits clarify when safety concerns override privacy protections while ensuring that crisis interventions comply with legal requirements and professional standards for information sharing and emergency intervention.

Informed consent addresses group members' understanding of crisis intervention procedures while ensuring that they are aware of circumstances that might require breach of confidentiality or emergency intervention.

Duty to warn obligations specify requirements for protecting potential victims of violence while balancing individual privacy rights with public safety responsibilities during crisis situations.

Involuntary commitment procedures outline legal requirements for emergency psychiatric evaluation while ensuring that these interventions are used appropriately and with proper legal authorization.

Documentation standards specify information that must be recorded to meet legal and regulatory requirements while protecting both patients and providers from liability related to crisis intervention decisions.

Incident Documentation

Accurate crisis documentation protects both patients and providers while meeting legal requirements and providing information necessary for quality improvement and risk management activities.

Objective description records factual information about crisis events while avoiding subjective interpretations or judgments that might not be supported by observable evidence.

Timeline documentation provides detailed chronology of crisis development and intervention while ensuring that decision-making processes and intervention rationales are clearly recorded.

Intervention justification explains the reasoning behind specific crisis interventions while demonstrating adherence to professional standards and evidence-based practices.

Outcome recording documents crisis resolution and ongoing safety planning while providing information necessary for follow-up care and treatment plan modifications.

Quality improvement uses crisis documentation to identify system improvements while protecting patient privacy and maintaining confidentiality of individual crisis events.

Training and Competency Development

Effective crisis management requires ongoing education and skill development while maintaining current knowledge about best practices and evidence-based interventions for various types of psychiatric emergencies.

Crisis intervention training provides specific skills for managing psychiatric emergencies while building confidence and competency in crisis assessment and intervention techniques.

Medical emergency preparedness ensures appropriate response to physical health crises while maintaining skills in basic life support and emergency medical response.

De-escalation techniques develop verbal and non-verbal communication skills while building ability to reduce tension and prevent crisis escalation through therapeutic intervention.

Legal education maintains current knowledge of regulatory requirements while understanding professional obligations and liability issues related to crisis intervention and emergency care.

Self-care planning addresses the emotional impact of crisis work while developing strategies for maintaining personal well-being and professional effectiveness despite exposure to traumatic situations.

Building Crisis Resilience

Effective crisis management builds both individual and group capacity for managing future emergencies while creating cultures of safety that support therapeutic risk-taking and emotional expression within appropriate boundaries.

Prevention focus addresses factors that contribute to crisis development while building individual and group skills for early intervention and crisis prevention rather than relying solely on emergency response.

Skill development teaches group members crisis management techniques while building their confidence and capacity for supporting each other during difficult situations.

Support network strengthening builds connections between group members while creating resources for ongoing mutual support that extends beyond formal group sessions.

Recovery planning addresses post-crisis treatment needs while ensuring that crisis experiences are integrated into ongoing therapeutic work rather than becoming sources of shame or treatment dropout.

Systemic improvement uses crisis experiences to strengthen organizational capacity while building systems that support both crisis prevention and effective emergency response.

Practice Wisdom

Crisis management in group settings represents one of the most challenging aspects of psychiatric nursing while offering opportunities for profound therapeutic growth and healing when handled skillfully and compassionately. Your ability to remain calm and therapeutic during emergencies provides essential modeling for group members while building their confidence in their own capacity for managing life crises.

The group setting provides unique opportunities for members to support each other through crises while building resilience and coping skills that serve them throughout their recovery journeys. Your role in facilitating these supportive responses while maintaining safety creates healing experiences that extend far beyond individual crisis resolution.

Emergency Management Essentials

- Environmental safety protocols require systematic attention to physical spaces and emergency preparedness while maintaining therapeutic atmosphere and accessibility
- Risk assessment procedures use standardized tools and clinical evaluation to identify individuals requiring additional safety support or modified interventions
- De-escalation scripts provide structured verbal interventions that reduce tension while maintaining therapeutic relationships and group safety
- Safety planning worksheets involve individuals in developing personalized crisis management strategies while building confidence and self-efficacy
- Emergency response protocols ensure appropriate responses to various crisis situations while maintaining clarity about roles and communication requirements
- Post-crisis debriefing provides learning opportunities while addressing emotional impact and identifying system improvements for future crisis prevention

Chapter 15: Program Development and Evaluation

The systematic development of group therapy programs requires a sophisticated understanding of organizational dynamics, resource allocation, outcome measurement, and continuous quality improvement that transforms individual therapeutic skills into sustainable programs serving multiple patients across extended timeframes. Program development represents the bridge between clinical expertise and administrative leadership that ensures effective group interventions reach the populations that need them most.

Your nursing education provides excellent foundation for program development because you understand healthcare systems, regulatory requirements, quality improvement processes, and the practical considerations that determine whether innovative programs succeed or fail in real-world healthcare environments.

Needs Assessment Strategies

Effective program development begins with systematic evaluation of community mental health needs, existing service gaps, and organizational capacity to deliver quality group interventions while ensuring that new programs address genuine needs rather than creating services for their own sake (30).

Community health assessment examines local mental health statistics, demographic trends, and service utilization patterns while identifying underserved populations and unmet treatment needs that could be addressed through group interventions.

Stakeholder analysis identifies key individuals and organizations whose support is necessary for program success while building understanding of political dynamics and resource allocation processes that influence program viability.

Gap analysis compares existing services with identified needs while highlighting specific areas where group interventions could provide effective, efficient treatment options that complement existing services.

Resource assessment evaluates available funding, staffing, space, and administrative support while building realistic understanding of organizational capacity for supporting new program development and implementation.

Regulatory review examines licensing requirements, accreditation standards, and legal obligations while ensuring that proposed programs comply with applicable regulations and professional standards.

Logic Models for Groups

Logic models provide systematic frameworks for planning group programs while articulating the theoretical connections between program activities, expected outcomes, and broader organizational goals that justify resource allocation and support.

Input identification specifies human resources, financial support, space requirements, and material needs while building comprehensive understanding of program resource requirements and implementation costs.

Activity planning details specific group interventions, session formats, duration, and intensity while ensuring that program activities align with identified needs and evidence-based practices.

Output measurement defines measurable products such as number of groups conducted, participants served, and sessions completed while establishing accountability mechanisms for tracking program implementation.

Outcome specification articulates expected changes in participant knowledge, skills, behavior, and clinical status while connecting group interventions to meaningful improvements in mental health and functioning.

Impact projection describes broader community benefits such as reduced healthcare utilization, improved quality of life, and cost savings while building support for program continuation and expansion.

Case Example: Developing Adolescent Depression Program

Our healthcare system identified adolescent depression as a significant community need requiring specialized group interventions that could provide effective treatment while managing cost constraints and integrating with existing services.

Needs assessment revealed that local emergency departments were seeing increasing numbers of depressed teenagers while outpatient providers had long waiting lists and limited experience with adolescent-specific interventions, creating gaps in accessible, age-appropriate treatment.

Stakeholder engagement involved school counselors, pediatricians, family advocates, and hospital administrators in program planning while building support coalition that could provide referrals, resources, and ongoing advocacy for program sustainability.

Evidence review examined research on adolescent depression group interventions while identifying specific approaches with strongest outcomes for teenage populations and adapting these models for local implementation.

Resource planning calculated costs for specialized staff training, adolescent-appropriate space modifications, family involvement components, and outcome measurement while developing realistic budget projections and funding strategies.

Implementation timeline established phases for staff recruitment and training, program marketing, initial group launches, and evaluation activities while building momentum for program success through careful sequencing of development activities.

The **pilot program** served 24 teenagers over six months while tracking clinical outcomes, participant satisfaction, family feedback, and staff experiences that informed program refinements and sustainability planning.

Outcome evaluation demonstrated significant improvements in depression scores, school functioning, and family relationships while documenting cost-effectiveness compared to individual therapy and emergency service utilization.

Program success led to **expansion planning** that included additional group formats, extended age ranges, and integration with school-based services while maintaining quality and effectiveness standards established during pilot implementation.

Budget Planning Worksheets

Systematic financial planning ensures program sustainability while providing accurate cost projections and resource allocation strategies that support quality programming within available budget constraints.

Personnel costs calculate salaries, benefits, and training expenses for group facilitators while accounting for preparation time, documentation requirements, and ongoing supervision needs that extend beyond direct service hours.

Facility expenses include space rental, utilities, maintenance, and insurance costs while considering special requirements for group rooms, privacy needs, and accessibility accommodations.

Material costs cover assessment instruments, therapeutic supplies, educational materials, and technology needs while planning for ongoing replacement and updating requirements.

Administrative overhead allocates costs for program management, marketing, quality assurance, and evaluation activities while ensuring adequate support for program operations and development.

Revenue projections estimate income from insurance reimbursement, grants, donations, and fee-for-service arrangements while building realistic financial models that support program sustainability.

Staffing Calculations

Appropriate staffing ensures quality group facilitation while managing costs and building sustainable programs that can recruit and retain qualified personnel over extended timeframes.

Facilitator requirements specify education, training, experience, and supervision needs while ensuring that group leaders have appropriate qualifications for specific populations and intervention approaches.

Support staff needs identify administrative, clinical, and technical personnel required for program operations while building comprehensive understanding of human resource requirements.

Training investments calculate costs for initial staff development and ongoing education while ensuring that facilitators maintain current knowledge and skills necessary for effective group leadership.

Supervision planning allocates time and resources for clinical oversight while ensuring that group facilitators receive appropriate guidance and support for managing complex clinical situations.

Recruitment strategies address challenges in finding qualified group facilitators while developing competitive compensation packages and professional development opportunities that attract excellent candidates.

Case Example: Implementing Dual Diagnosis Program

Our community mental health center needed to develop dual diagnosis groups serving individuals with co-occurring mental health and substance use disorders while coordinating with addiction treatment providers and managing complex regulatory requirements.

Program planning involved extensive collaboration with addiction counselors, psychiatrists, and regulatory agencies while building understanding of integrated treatment approaches and compliance requirements for serving dual diagnosis populations.

Staff development required specialized training in integrated treatment models while building competencies in both mental health and addiction interventions that could be delivered effectively in group formats.

Space requirements included consideration of stigma reduction, accessibility for individuals with various disabilities, and coordination with existing addiction services while creating welcoming environments for this vulnerable population.

Outcome measurement addressed both mental health and substance use indicators while building comprehensive evaluation systems that could demonstrate effectiveness to multiple funding sources and regulatory agencies.

Sustainability planning developed diversified funding strategies while building partnerships with addiction treatment providers that could support ongoing program operations and participant recruitment.

The **implementation process** served 48 individuals over the first year while tracking clinical outcomes, treatment retention, and cost-effectiveness compared to traditional sequential treatment approaches.

Quality improvement addressed initial challenges with group attendance, staff coordination, and outcome measurement while making program modifications that improved effectiveness and participant satisfaction.

Program success demonstrated the value of integrated approaches while providing model for replication in other communities and building support for expansion to additional populations and service locations.

Case Example: Geriatric Mental Health Program Development

Our healthcare system recognized growing need for geriatric mental health services as the community aged while existing providers lacked specialized knowledge and geriatric-appropriate interventions.

Demographic analysis revealed rapidly increasing older adult population with high rates of depression, anxiety, and social isolation while existing services were designed primarily for younger adults and lacked geriatric expertise.

Service gap identification showed that older adults had difficulty accessing mental health services due to transportation barriers, stigma about mental health treatment, and provider inexperience with geriatric presentations.

Evidence-based planning incorporated research on effective group interventions for older adults while adapting approaches for cognitive changes, sensory impairments, and medical comorbidities common in this population.

Facility modifications addressed accessibility requirements, lighting needs, acoustic considerations, and comfort factors while creating environments that supported successful participation by older adults with various physical limitations.

Family involvement planned for adult children and spouse participation while addressing complex family dynamics and caregiving responsibilities that affect treatment engagement and outcomes.

The **program launch** included reminiscence therapy groups, anxiety management groups, and grief support groups while tracking participation patterns, clinical outcomes, and family satisfaction with services.

Community partnership development connected the program with senior centers, primary care providers, and social services while building referral networks and support systems for ongoing program success.

Outcome evaluation demonstrated improvements in depression, social engagement, and quality of life while documenting reduced healthcare utilization and increased family satisfaction with mental health services.

Space and Resource Requirements

Physical environments significantly affect group dynamics and therapeutic outcomes while requiring careful planning that balances therapeutic needs with cost constraints and practical considerations.

Room specifications address size requirements for different group formats while ensuring adequate space for movement, comfort, and privacy that supports therapeutic engagement and safety.

Furniture selection provides comfortable, supportive seating arranged to promote interaction while accommodating individuals with mobility limitations and creating welcoming, non-institutional atmospheres.

Technology integration includes audio-visual equipment, communication devices, and telehealth capabilities while ensuring that technology supports rather than interferes with therapeutic relationships and group processes.

Storage needs accommodate therapeutic materials, assessment instruments, and personal belongings while maintaining organization and security necessary for effective program operations.

Accessibility compliance ensures that facilities meet requirements for individuals with disabilities while creating universally accessible environments that welcome all potential participants.

Continuous Quality Improvement

Systematic quality improvement processes ensure that group programs maintain effectiveness while adapting to changing needs and incorporating new evidence-based practices that improve outcomes and participant satisfaction.

Outcome monitoring tracks clinical indicators, participant satisfaction, and program metrics while identifying trends and patterns that inform program modifications and quality enhancement activities.

Process evaluation examines program implementation while identifying operational improvements that could increase efficiency, effectiveness, or participant engagement with services.

Participant feedback incorporates group member perspectives while building understanding of program strengths and areas needing improvement from the consumer perspective.

Staff input utilizes facilitator observations and recommendations while building organizational learning that improves program quality and staff satisfaction with their work.

External evaluation seeks objective assessment from independent reviewers while gaining perspectives that internal evaluation might miss due to organizational bias or limited viewpoints.

Sustainability Planning

Long-term program success requires systematic planning for financial sustainability, staff retention, and organizational support that extends beyond initial funding periods and founding leadership transitions.

Diversified funding develops multiple revenue sources while reducing dependence on single funding streams that might disappear due to policy changes or economic fluctuations.

Outcome documentation provides evidence for continued funding while demonstrating program value to stakeholders and decision-makers who control resource allocation.

Staff development builds internal capacity while reducing dependence on external consultants and creating organizational knowledge that survives personnel changes.

Community integration establishes program connections with local organizations while building political support and community ownership that supports ongoing program survival.

Succession planning prepares for leadership transitions while ensuring that program knowledge and relationships survive changes in key personnel.

Marketing and Outreach

Effective programs require comprehensive marketing strategies that reach appropriate populations while building community awareness and support for group mental health services.

Target audience identification specifies demographic characteristics and communication preferences while developing culturally appropriate outreach strategies that resonate with intended participants.

Message development creates compelling communications while addressing stigma and misconceptions about mental health treatment that might prevent service utilization.

Communication channels utilize appropriate media and community connections while reaching target populations through trusted sources and familiar venues.

Professional education informs referral sources while building provider knowledge about group interventions and appropriate referral criteria.

Community engagement participates in health fairs, educational events, and community organizations while building relationships that support ongoing program visibility and referrals.

Program Evaluation Methods

Systematic evaluation provides evidence for program effectiveness while identifying areas for improvement and building support for continued funding and organizational commitment.

Quantitative measures track clinical outcomes, participation rates, and cost-effectiveness while providing objective data about program performance and participant improvement.

Qualitative assessment captures participant experiences, staff observations, and family feedback while building understanding of program impact that numbers alone cannot convey.

Comparison studies evaluate program outcomes against control groups or alternative treatments while building evidence for group intervention effectiveness and value.

Long-term follow-up tracks participant outcomes after program completion while demonstrating sustained benefits and identifying factors that support ongoing recovery and well-being.

Cost-benefit analysis compares program costs with healthcare savings and quality of life improvements while building economic arguments for program continuation and expansion.

Innovation and Adaptation

Successful programs remain current with emerging research and changing community needs while adapting services to improve effectiveness and reach new populations that could benefit from group interventions.

Research integration incorporates new evidence-based practices while maintaining program fidelity to proven approaches that form the foundation of effective group treatment.

Technology adoption utilizes emerging technologies while ensuring that innovations support rather than replace human therapeutic relationships that remain central to group healing.

Population expansion adapts successful programs for new demographic groups while maintaining quality and effectiveness standards established in original program development.

Service integration coordinates with other healthcare services while building comprehensive treatment approaches that address complex needs requiring multiple interventions.

Dissemination planning shares successful program models while building capacity for replication in other communities and healthcare systems.

Program development represents the intersection of clinical expertise and organizational leadership that transforms individual therapeutic skills into sustainable services reaching multiple individuals over extended timeframes. Your nursing background provides excellent foundation for this work while requiring additional skills in project management, financial planning, and organizational development.

The investment required for effective program development pays dividends through improved patient outcomes, cost-effective service delivery, and enhanced organizational capacity for addressing community mental health needs through evidence-based group interventions.

Program Building Blocks

- Needs assessment strategies provide foundation for program development through systematic evaluation of community needs, service gaps, and organizational capacity
- Logic models articulate connections between program activities and expected outcomes while building support for resource allocation and program implementation
- Budget planning worksheets ensure financial sustainability through accurate cost projections and revenue planning that support quality programming
- Staffing calculations determine appropriate personnel requirements while ensuring qualified facilitation and adequate supervision for effective group leadership
- Continuous quality improvement maintains program effectiveness through systematic monitoring and adaptation based on outcome data and participant feedback
- Sustainability planning ensures long-term program success through diversified funding, community integration, and organizational capacity building

Chapter 16: Psychoeducational Groups for Specific Disorders

The art of teaching complex psychiatric concepts to individuals experiencing the very symptoms you're explaining requires a unique blend of clinical knowledge, educational skill, and therapeutic sensitivity that transforms medical information into healing experiences. Psychoeducational groups bridge the gap between what patients need to know about their conditions and what they can actually absorb and apply while managing symptoms that often interfere with learning, memory, and concentration.

Your nursing expertise provides distinct advantages in disorder-specific education because you understand how symptoms affect cognitive functioning, how medications influence learning capacity, and how to adapt teaching methods for individuals whose psychiatric conditions create barriers to traditional educational approaches. You also recognize that knowledge alone rarely changes behavior—effective psychoeducation must connect information to personal experience while building motivation for self-care and recovery.

Depression Education Groups

Depression education groups address the widespread misconceptions about depressive disorders while providing practical information that helps participants understand their condition as medical illness requiring appropriate treatment rather than personal weakness or character flaw (31).

Symptom education explains how depression affects thinking, emotions, behavior, and physical functioning while helping participants recognize that their experiences represent legitimate medical symptoms rather than personal failures or lack of willpower.

Brain chemistry basics describes how neurotransmitter imbalances contribute to depressive symptoms while providing scientific foundation that reduces stigma and builds understanding of why medications and therapy are necessary rather than optional treatments.

Treatment options overview covers various approaches including medications, psychotherapy, and lifestyle modifications while helping participants understand that effective depression treatment often requires multiple interventions working together over extended timeframes.

Recovery timelines prepare participants for the reality that depression treatment typically requires weeks or months to show significant improvement while preventing premature treatment discontinuation when progress feels slow or minimal.

Relapse prevention teaches participants to recognize early warning signs of depression recurrence while developing strategies for maintaining wellness and seeking help promptly when symptoms begin to return.

Case Example: Depression Education for Postpartum Group

Our postpartum depression education group addressed the unique challenges facing eight new mothers whose depression was complicated by hormonal changes, sleep deprivation, and societal expectations about maternal joy and bonding.

Sarah, a 29-year-old first-time mother, exemplified common misconceptions about postpartum depression. She believed her symptoms indicated that she was a "bad mother" and feared that seeking help would result in losing custody of her infant daughter.

Hormone education helped Sarah understand how dramatic hormonal shifts after childbirth contribute to depression while normalizing her experience as medical condition rather than maternal inadequacy or personal weakness.

The group learned about **prevalence statistics** showing that postpartum depression affects up to 20% of new mothers while building understanding that this condition is common rather than rare or shameful experience.

Risk factor discussion covered biological vulnerabilities, social stressors, and psychological factors that increase postpartum depression risk while helping participants understand multiple contributors rather than blaming themselves for their conditions.

Treatment safety addressed concerns about breastfeeding while taking antidepressant medications, providing evidence-based information about medication safety while supporting informed decision-making about treatment options.

Support system building taught participants how to communicate their needs to partners and family members while building networks that could provide practical assistance and emotional support during recovery.

Sarah's transformation through education demonstrated the power of accurate information in reducing shame and building treatment motivation. Her depression scores improved significantly as she developed understanding of her condition and confidence in treatment approaches.

Anxiety and Panic Disorder Groups

Anxiety education groups address the high prevalence of anxiety disorders while providing information that helps participants understand the difference between normal worry and pathological anxiety requiring professional treatment.

Anxiety types differentiation explains various anxiety disorders including generalized anxiety, panic disorder, social anxiety, and specific phobias while helping participants identify their specific presentations and appropriate treatment approaches.

Fight-or-flight education describes the physiological basis of anxiety responses while helping participants understand that anxiety symptoms represent normal bodily functions that have become overactive rather than dangerous or life-threatening experiences.

Panic attack demystification provides detailed explanation of panic symptoms while teaching participants that panic attacks, though uncomfortable, are not dangerous and will end naturally without causing physical harm.

Avoidance cycle explanation shows how avoiding anxiety-provoking situations actually increases anxiety over time while building motivation for exposure-based treatments that gradually reduce anxiety through facing feared situations.

Coping skills instruction teaches specific techniques for managing anxiety including breathing exercises, progressive muscle relaxation, and cognitive restructuring while providing tools that participants can use immediately to improve their symptoms.

Case Example: Panic Disorder Education for Workplace Group

Our workplace-based panic disorder education group served twelve employees whose panic attacks were interfering with job performance and creating fears about career security and professional competence.

Michael, a 34-year-old accountant, had experienced multiple panic attacks during important meetings, leading to avoidance of presentations and declining job performance that threatened his career advancement.

Panic symptom education helped Michael understand that his racing heart, sweating, and feelings of impending doom represented anxiety responses rather than heart attacks or professional incompetence that he had feared.

The group learned **workplace triggers** identification while developing strategies for managing anxiety in professional settings without drawing unwanted attention or compromising job performance.

Accommodation discussion covered Americans with Disabilities Act protections while building understanding of rights and resources available for managing mental health conditions in workplace settings.

Disclosure decisions addressed the complex considerations involved in telling supervisors or colleagues about panic disorder while respecting individual preferences about privacy and professional reputation.

Success strategies included practical techniques for managing panic symptoms during meetings, presentations, and other work-related activities while building confidence in participants' ability to maintain successful careers despite anxiety disorders.

Michael's improvement through education and peer support allowed him to return to full job participation while developing strategies for managing anxiety that enhanced rather than hindered his professional performance.

Bipolar Disorder Management Groups

Bipolar disorder education addresses the complexity of mood disorders while providing information that helps participants understand their condition as chronic illness requiring ongoing management rather than episodic problem requiring only crisis intervention.

Mood cycle education explains the patterns of manic, hypomanic, and depressive episodes while helping participants recognize early warning signs that can guide early intervention and prevention strategies.

Medication importance addresses the necessity of mood stabilizers for preventing episodes while building understanding of why medication adherence is essential even during periods of mood stability.

Lifestyle factors cover sleep hygiene, stress management, substance avoidance, and routine maintenance while teaching participants how daily choices affect mood stability and episode risk.

Episode management provides strategies for coping with breakthrough symptoms while building skills for maintaining safety and functioning during periods of mood instability.

Long-term planning addresses career, relationship, and life goal considerations while helping participants develop realistic expectations and strategies for achieving meaningful lives despite bipolar disorder.

Case Example: Bipolar Education for College Students

Our bipolar disorder education group for college students addressed the unique challenges of managing this condition during a life stage characterized by irregular schedules, academic stress, and social pressures that can trigger mood episodes.

Jessica, a 20-year-old junior, had experienced her first manic episode during sophomore year, resulting in academic probation and social difficulties that she struggled to understand and manage.

College-specific triggers education helped Jessica identify how sleep deprivation, academic stress, and social drinking could precipitate mood episodes while developing strategies for managing these common college experiences safely.

The group learned **academic accommodations** available through disability services while building understanding of how to access support without stigma or academic penalty.

Social challenges discussion addressed how to maintain friendships while managing bipolar disorder, including disclosure decisions and strategies for participating in social activities without compromising mood stability.

Career planning helped participants consider how bipolar disorder might affect their professional goals while developing strategies for building successful careers that accommodate their mental health needs.

Family communication addressed the complex dynamics of young adult independence while maintaining family support for mental health management during the college years.

Jessica's education group participation helped her develop realistic strategies for completing college successfully while learning to manage bipolar disorder as ongoing health condition rather than temporary crisis.

Schizophrenia and Psychosis Education Groups

Schizophrenia education groups address the widespread misconceptions about psychotic disorders while providing information that helps participants and their families understand these conditions as brain disorders requiring medical treatment and social support.

Symptom explanation covers positive symptoms (hallucinations, delusions), negative symptoms (social withdrawal, reduced motivation), and cognitive symptoms (memory, attention problems) while building understanding of the complex nature of schizophrenia spectrum disorders.

Brain disease education explains the neurobiological basis of schizophrenia while reducing stigma through scientific understanding of these conditions as medical disorders rather than personal choices or character flaws.

Medication education addresses the necessity of antipsychotic medications while providing information about side effects, monitoring requirements, and strategies for maximizing benefits while minimizing adverse effects.

Recovery orientation builds hope through discussion of recovery possibilities while acknowledging the chronic nature of these conditions and the importance of ongoing treatment and support.

Family involvement recognizes the crucial role of family support while providing education about how families can best help their relatives manage these challenging conditions.

PTSD and Trauma Groups

Trauma education groups address the complex effects of traumatic experiences while providing information that helps participants understand their symptoms as normal responses to abnormal situations rather than personal weakness or mental illness.

Trauma response education explains how the brain and body respond to life-threatening experiences while normalizing symptoms such as hypervigilance, nightmares, and emotional numbing as adaptive responses that can become problematic over time.

PTSD symptom clusters cover re-experiencing, avoidance, negative alterations in mood and cognition, and arousal symptoms while helping participants recognize their experiences as part of identifiable medical condition with effective treatments.

Recovery possibilities build hope through discussion of evidence-based treatments while acknowledging that trauma recovery is possible with appropriate help and support.

Safety planning addresses ongoing safety concerns while building skills for managing triggers and symptoms in daily life situations that might activate trauma responses.

Support system development helps participants build networks of understanding friends and family while reducing isolation that often accompanies trauma experiences.

Case Example: PTSD Education for Veterans Group

Our veterans' PTSD education group addressed the unique challenges facing eight military veterans whose combat trauma was complicated by military culture, reintegration difficulties, and barriers to seeking mental health treatment.

Robert, a 28-year-old Marine veteran, had experienced multiple combat deployments and struggled with nightmares, hypervigilance, and angry outbursts that were affecting his relationships and employment.

Military culture discussion addressed how military training and culture could both contribute to PTSD symptoms and create barriers to seeking help while building understanding of the unique aspects of military trauma.

The group learned about **moral injury** as distinct from PTSD while building understanding of how actions during combat might create different types of psychological wounds requiring different healing approaches.

Civilian reintegration education addressed the challenges of transitioning from military to civilian life while building understanding of how these transitions could complicate trauma recovery.

Family impact discussion covered how PTSD affects spouses and children while providing strategies for maintaining relationships and building family support for recovery efforts.

Career considerations addressed how PTSD might affect employment while building strategies for job success and disclosure decisions that protected both recovery and professional advancement.

Robert's group participation helped him understand his symptoms as normal responses to abnormal combat experiences while building motivation for treatment and strategies for successful civilian reintegration.

Personality Disorder Skills Training

Personality disorder education groups focus on skill development rather than pathology while providing information that helps participants understand their conditions as patterns that can be modified through sustained effort and appropriate interventions.

Pattern recognition helps participants identify recurring themes in their relationships and behaviors while building awareness that can support positive change efforts.

Skill deficits identification addresses areas such as emotion regulation, interpersonal effectiveness, and distress tolerance while building understanding of specific abilities that can be developed through practice.

Treatment approaches cover evidence-based interventions such as dialectical behavior therapy and cognitive-behavioral therapy while building realistic expectations about treatment length and requirements.

Recovery orientation focuses on growth possibilities while acknowledging the persistent nature of personality patterns and the sustained effort required for meaningful change.

Relationship skills address the interpersonal difficulties common in personality disorders while providing concrete strategies for building and maintaining healthier relationships.

Adapting Teaching Methods for Symptoms

Effective psychoeducation requires modification of teaching approaches based on how psychiatric symptoms affect learning capacity while ensuring that information remains accessible despite cognitive, emotional, or behavioral barriers to traditional education.

Attention accommodation addresses how depression, anxiety, and psychosis affect concentration while using shorter segments, frequent breaks, and multiple modalities to maintain engagement.

Memory support provides written materials, repetition, and review activities while accommodating the memory difficulties common in many psychiatric conditions.

Anxiety management creates safe learning environments while using gradual exposure and choice-based participation that reduces anxiety about learning new information.

Cognitive adaptation simplifies complex concepts while using concrete examples and visual aids that support understanding despite cognitive impairment or processing difficulties.

Motivation building connects information to personal goals while addressing the apathy and hopelessness that can interfere with learning motivation in many psychiatric conditions.

Case Example: Adapting Education for Cognitive Impairment

Our schizophrenia education group required significant adaptations to accommodate the cognitive symptoms that affected participants' ability to process and retain information about their condition and treatment.

David, a 32-year-old with schizophrenia, demonstrated typical cognitive challenges including attention difficulties, memory problems, and processing speed limitations that interfered with traditional educational approaches.

Simplified language replaced medical terminology with everyday words while maintaining accuracy and avoiding condescending communication that could undermine therapeutic relationships.

Visual aids included diagrams, charts, and pictures that supported verbal information while accommodating different learning styles and cognitive processing preferences.

Repetition strategies presented key concepts multiple times in different formats while providing frequent review and practice opportunities that supported retention.

Interactive methods engaged multiple senses while using hands-on activities that maintained attention and supported learning despite concentration difficulties.

Paced delivery allowed adequate processing time while avoiding information overload that could overwhelm cognitive capacity and interfere with comprehension.

David's progress through adapted education demonstrated the importance of matching teaching methods to cognitive abilities while maintaining respect and therapeutic value despite necessary modifications.

Measuring Knowledge Acquisition

Systematic assessment of learning outcomes ensures that psychoeducational groups achieve their intended goals while identifying participants who need additional support or different educational approaches.

Pre-post testing measures knowledge changes while providing objective data about educational effectiveness and participant learning.

Skill demonstration evaluates practical application while ensuring that information translates into behavioral changes that support recovery goals.

Retention assessment measures long-term learning while identifying information that may need reinforcement or different presentation methods.

Satisfaction evaluation captures participant perspectives while building understanding of educational approaches that feel most helpful and engaging.

Behavioral outcomes track real-world application while measuring whether increased knowledge leads to improved self-care and treatment engagement.

Cultural Adaptations for Education

Psychoeducational content must be adapted for diverse cultural backgrounds while respecting different beliefs about mental illness and ensuring that information feels relevant and acceptable to various populations.

Language considerations address both literal translation needs and cultural concepts that may not have direct equivalents while ensuring accurate communication across linguistic differences.

Cultural beliefs integration acknowledges traditional healing practices while building bridges between cultural wisdom and modern psychiatric understanding.

Family involvement adaptation respects different cultural patterns of family decision-making while ensuring that education reaches appropriate family members and community supports.

Stigma sensitivity addresses how different cultures view mental illness while providing education that reduces rather than increases stigma and shame.

Community resources connect participants with culturally appropriate support services while building understanding of available resources that honor cultural preferences and values.

Technology Integration

Modern psychoeducational groups increasingly incorporate technology components that can enhance learning while accommodating different learning styles and providing resources that extend beyond formal group sessions.

Digital resources supplement in-person education while providing access to additional information and support that participants can access as needed.

Interactive applications engage participants actively while using gaming elements and multimedia presentations that appeal to different learning preferences.

Virtual reality provides immersive experiences while offering exposure opportunities and skill practice in controlled environments that feel safe and supportive.

Mobile apps extend learning beyond group sessions while providing ongoing reinforcement and support for applying educational content in daily life.

Online communities connect participants with others facing similar challenges while building support networks that complement formal educational programming.

Building Treatment Motivation

Effective psychoeducation goes beyond information delivery to build genuine motivation for engaging in treatment while addressing ambivalence and resistance that often accompany psychiatric conditions.

Personal relevance connects medical information to individual experiences while helping participants understand how education applies to their specific situations and goals.

Hope building demonstrates recovery possibilities while providing realistic expectations about treatment outcomes and recovery processes.

Choice emphasis respects autonomy while providing information that supports informed decision-making about treatment options and life choices.

Strength identification recognizes existing resources while building confidence in participants' capacity for managing their conditions and achieving their goals.

Peer support harnesses shared experiences while creating communities that reinforce educational messages and support sustained behavior change.

Moving Forward with Knowledge

Psychoeducational groups represent the foundation upon which all other therapeutic interventions build—without accurate understanding of their conditions, participants cannot make informed decisions about treatment or develop realistic expectations about recovery processes. Your role as educator and healer positions you to provide this foundation while building therapeutic relationships that support sustained engagement with treatment.

The knowledge participants gain through disorder-specific education becomes the lens through which they view their experiences and make decisions about their care. This perspective shapes not only their immediate treatment engagement but their long-term relationship with their mental health and recovery journey.

Educational Foundations

- Depression education groups reduce stigma through brain chemistry basics while building understanding of treatment necessity and recovery timelines
- Anxiety and panic disorder education demystifies symptoms while teaching participants that anxiety responses are not dangerous and can be managed effectively

- Bipolar disorder management education addresses the chronic nature requiring ongoing treatment while building skills for episode prevention and lifestyle management
- Schizophrenia and psychosis education reduces stigma through scientific understanding while building hope through recovery-oriented information and family involvement
- PTSD and trauma education normalizes symptoms as responses to abnormal situations while building safety skills and support system development
- Teaching method adaptations accommodate cognitive, emotional, and behavioral symptoms while ensuring information accessibility despite psychiatric barriers to learning

Chapter 17: Integrating Groups with Nursing Care Plans

The seamless integration of group therapy participation with individual nursing care plans represents one of the most sophisticated aspects of psychiatric nursing practice, requiring you to synthesize group observations with individual assessments while coordinating care across multiple providers and treatment modalities. This integration ensures that group experiences contribute meaningfully to each participant's unique recovery goals rather than existing as isolated treatment components disconnected from overall care planning.

Your nursing expertise in care plan development provides distinct advantages for this integration because you understand how to translate group participation into measurable outcomes, document therapeutic progress across multiple domains, and communicate effectively with interdisciplinary teams about both individual and group-level interventions and their impact on patient care.

Care Plan Integration Strategies

Effective integration requires systematic approaches that connect group participation goals with individual treatment objectives while ensuring that both individual and group interventions work synergistically to support each patient's recovery process (32).

Goal alignment ensures that group therapy objectives directly support individual care plan goals while avoiding conflicts between group expectations and personalized treatment priorities that could confuse or overwhelm patients.

Outcome measurement consistency uses the same assessment tools and criteria for both individual and group progress while providing coherent evaluation systems that track improvement across all treatment modalities.

Documentation coordination creates unified records that capture both individual responses to group participation and group-level dynamics that influence individual progress while maintaining comprehensive treatment records.

Treatment team communication establishes protocols for sharing group observations with individual providers while ensuring that all team members understand how group participation supports overall treatment goals and recovery planning.

Intervention sequencing coordinates the timing of individual and group interventions while building treatment progression that maximizes the benefits of both modalities through careful integration rather than parallel delivery.

Case Example: Integrating Depression Group with Individual Care Plans

Our inpatient depression unit developed systematic approaches for integrating group therapy participation with individual nursing care plans for twelve patients whose treatment required coordination across multiple therapeutic modalities and provider disciplines.

Maria, a 42-year-old patient with major depressive disorder, exemplified the complexity of integration challenges. Her individual care plan addressed medication adherence, safety monitoring, and family relationship improvement while her group therapy focused on cognitive restructuring and peer support development.

Care plan modification incorporated specific group therapy goals including "patient will practice challenging negative thoughts in group settings" and "patient will provide peer support to other group members" while connecting these objectives to her individual goals for improved mood and social functioning.

Progress documentation tracked Maria's group participation using standardized assessment tools that measured both her individual therapeutic progress and her contributions to group therapeutic factors such as hope instillation and universality.

Provider communication included weekly interdisciplinary meetings where group therapy observations were shared with psychiatrists, social workers, and individual therapists while building comprehensive understanding of Maria's progress across all treatment modalities.

Discharge planning incorporated group therapy insights about Maria's social skills, peer relationships, and coping strategies while developing community referrals and ongoing support plans that built upon her group therapy gains.

Family involvement used information from group therapy about Maria's communication patterns and relationship skills while developing family therapy goals and interventions that reinforced her group therapy learning.

Maria's integrated treatment demonstrated significant improvements in depression scores, social functioning, and treatment engagement while showing how group participation enhanced rather than competed with individual therapeutic interventions.

Documentation Systems

Systematic documentation captures the complex interactions between individual patient needs and group therapeutic processes while meeting regulatory requirements and supporting quality improvement initiatives.

Individual progress notes document each patient's group participation while recording specific behaviors, therapeutic responses, and progress toward individual care plan goals that can be observed and measured within group settings.

Group summary reports capture overall group dynamics and therapeutic factors while identifying patterns and trends that might affect individual patient progress or suggest modifications to group interventions.

Critical incident documentation records significant events during group sessions while describing their impact on individual participants and documenting appropriate interventions and follow-up care provided.

Outcome tracking systems measure both individual patient progress and group-level outcomes while providing data for quality improvement initiatives and evidence-based practice development.

Treatment team records document communication between group facilitators and other providers while ensuring that group observations inform broader treatment planning and care coordination efforts.

Case Example: Documentation for Dual Diagnosis Integration

Our dual diagnosis unit required sophisticated documentation systems that captured the complex interactions between mental health and substance use treatment while integrating group therapy observations with individual addiction counseling and psychiatric care.

James, a 35-year-old patient with bipolar disorder and alcohol use disorder, participated in multiple group interventions including mood management, addiction recovery, and dual diagnosis education while receiving individual therapy and psychiatric medication management.

Cross-system documentation tracked James's progress across both mental health and addiction treatment domains while using standardized assessment tools that measured integrated outcomes rather than separate conditions.

Provider communication logs documented regular communication between group facilitators, addiction counselors, and psychiatrists while ensuring that all providers understood how group participation affected both mood stability and substance use recovery.

Safety monitoring included protocols for documenting substance use disclosures during group sessions while ensuring appropriate follow-up and coordination with addiction treatment providers.

Treatment planning integration used group therapy observations to inform individual addiction counseling goals while incorporating substance use recovery milestones into group therapy progress tracking.

Discharge coordination combined insights from all group and individual providers while developing comprehensive continuing care plans that addressed both mental health and substance use recovery needs.

James's integrated documentation demonstrated the complexity of dual diagnosis treatment while showing how systematic record-keeping supported effective care coordination and improved treatment outcomes.

Interdisciplinary Communication

Effective integration requires sophisticated communication systems that ensure all treatment team members understand how group therapy participation affects individual patient progress while building collaborative approaches to complex care planning.

Team meeting protocols establish regular communication schedules while ensuring that group therapy observations are incorporated into treatment planning discussions and care plan modifications.

Communication templates provide structured formats for sharing group therapy information while ensuring consistent reporting of relevant observations and therapeutic progress across different providers.

Role clarification defines responsibilities for different team members while preventing duplication of efforts and ensuring that all aspects of integrated care are appropriately covered and coordinated.

Conflict resolution procedures address disagreements between providers while maintaining focus on patient welfare and evidence-based treatment approaches that support integrated care planning.

Outcome sharing ensures that all team members understand patient progress while building collective understanding of treatment effectiveness and areas needing additional attention or intervention.

Case Example: Interdisciplinary Integration for Trauma Recovery

Our trauma recovery program required extensive interdisciplinary coordination between group therapy facilitators, individual trauma therapists, psychiatrists, and social workers while ensuring that all interventions supported rather than hindered trauma recovery processes.

Susan, a 29-year-old survivor of childhood sexual abuse, participated in trauma-focused group therapy while receiving individual EMDR therapy and psychiatric medication management for PTSD and depression.

Treatment sequencing coordinated the timing of group and individual trauma processing while ensuring that group participation supported rather than overwhelmed Susan's capacity for trauma work in individual sessions.

Safety planning involved all team members in developing crisis intervention strategies while ensuring consistent responses to trauma reactions that might occur during any treatment modality.

Progress coordination shared observations about Susan's trauma recovery across all providers while building comprehensive understanding of her healing process and treatment responses.

Family therapy integration coordinated group therapy insights about Susan's relationship patterns with family therapy goals while ensuring that all interventions supported her recovery from childhood trauma.

Community referral planning used information from all treatment modalities while developing connections to trauma survivor support groups and community resources that could support long-term recovery.

Susan's integrated treatment demonstrated significant improvements in PTSD symptoms, relationship functioning, and overall life satisfaction while showing the importance of coordinated care for complex trauma presentations.

Outcome Tracking Across Settings

Systematic outcome measurement ensures that the benefits of integrated treatment can be documented and evaluated while providing evidence for the effectiveness of group therapy integration with individual care planning.

Standardized assessments measure patient progress using validated instruments while providing consistent outcome data that can be compared across different treatment modalities and settings.

Functional measures evaluate real-world improvements in daily living skills, social functioning, and quality of life while demonstrating the practical benefits of integrated treatment approaches.

Treatment satisfaction captures patient perspectives on integrated care while building understanding of which aspects of coordinated treatment feel most helpful and supportive.

Provider satisfaction evaluates staff experiences with integrated treatment while identifying system improvements that could enhance care coordination and communication effectiveness.

Cost-effectiveness analysis measures the economic benefits of integrated approaches while demonstrating value to healthcare systems and insurance providers who fund complex treatment programs.

Technology Support for Integration

Modern healthcare systems increasingly rely on technology platforms that support integrated care planning while providing communication tools and documentation systems that streamline coordination efforts.

Electronic health records provide platforms for integrated documentation while ensuring that all providers have access to current information about patient progress and treatment plans.

Communication systems facilitate secure messaging between providers while supporting real-time communication about patient needs and treatment coordination requirements.

Outcome tracking software automates data collection while providing dashboards and reports that help providers monitor patient progress and identify areas needing attention.

Scheduling coordination ensures that group and individual appointments are coordinated while avoiding conflicts and supporting patient attendance at all treatment modalities.

Quality assurance tools monitor compliance with integrated treatment protocols while identifying opportunities for system improvements and provider education.

Addressing Integration Challenges

Complex integrated treatment creates unique challenges that require systematic approaches and organizational commitment to overcome barriers that might interfere with effective care coordination.

Provider communication barriers can interfere with information sharing while requiring systematic solutions such as regular meetings, clear protocols, and shared documentation systems.

Scheduling conflicts between group and individual appointments can reduce treatment participation while requiring flexible scheduling and coordination between providers.

Conflicting treatment approaches may emerge when different providers have varying therapeutic orientations while requiring clear treatment protocols and regular communication to resolve differences.

Documentation burden can overwhelm providers while requiring efficient systems and shared responsibilities that reduce paperwork while maintaining quality records.

Resource limitations may constrain integrated treatment while requiring creative solutions and advocacy for adequate staffing and system support.

Quality Improvement Initiatives

Continuous improvement of integrated treatment requires systematic evaluation and modification of care coordination processes while building organizational capacity for effective interdisciplinary collaboration.

Process evaluation examines how well integration protocols work while identifying barriers and facilitators that affect care coordination effectiveness.

Outcome analysis measures the benefits of integrated treatment while comparing outcomes to non-integrated approaches and identifying areas for improvement.

Staff feedback incorporates provider perspectives while building understanding of system strengths and challenges from the perspective of those delivering coordinated care.

Patient input captures consumer perspectives while ensuring that integrated treatment approaches meet patient needs and preferences for coordinated care.

System modifications implement improvements based on evaluation findings while building organizational learning and capacity for effective integrated treatment delivery.

Training and Development

Successful integration requires ongoing education and skill development for all providers involved in coordinated care while building organizational competencies that support effective interdisciplinary collaboration.

Integration skills training teaches providers how to coordinate care effectively while building competencies in communication, documentation, and collaborative treatment planning.

Communication workshops develop skills for interdisciplinary collaboration while addressing common barriers and building effective working relationships across provider disciplines.

Documentation training ensures consistent and effective record-keeping while reducing burden and improving information sharing across treatment team members.

Quality improvement education builds understanding of continuous improvement processes while engaging providers in efforts to enhance integrated treatment effectiveness.

Leadership development prepares providers for coordination roles while building organizational capacity for managing complex integrated treatment programs.

Sustainability and Growth

Long-term success of integrated treatment approaches requires organizational commitment and system development that extends beyond individual provider enthusiasm to include administrative support and resource allocation.

Administrative support ensures adequate resources and organizational commitment while providing leadership necessary for sustained integrated treatment program success.

Financial planning addresses the costs of coordinated care while demonstrating value and building sustainable funding for integrated treatment approaches.

Expansion planning builds capacity for serving additional patients while maintaining quality and effectiveness standards established in initial integration efforts.

Research and evaluation documents outcomes and best practices while contributing to the evidence base for integrated treatment approaches and their benefits.

Dissemination activities share successful models while building capacity for integrated treatment replication in other healthcare systems and communities.

The integration of group therapy with individual nursing care plans represents the future of psychiatric nursing practice—moving beyond fragmented treatment approaches toward coordinated care that maximizes therapeutic benefits while reducing costs and improving patient satisfaction. Your role in developing and implementing these integrated approaches positions you at the forefront of healthcare innovation.

The patients you serve deserve treatment that addresses their needs holistically rather than through disconnected interventions that may work at cross-purposes. Integration ensures that every therapeutic contact builds upon previous interventions while contributing to comprehensive recovery plans that address the full spectrum of mental health needs.

Integration Essentials

- Care plan integration strategies align group therapy objectives with individual treatment goals while ensuring synergistic rather than competing interventions
- Documentation systems capture complex interactions between individual and group progress while meeting regulatory requirements and supporting quality improvement
- Interdisciplinary communication protocols ensure all team members understand how group participation affects individual progress while building collaborative treatment approaches
- Outcome tracking across settings provides evidence for integrated treatment effectiveness while identifying areas for improvement and system enhancement
- Technology support streamlines documentation and communication while providing tools that facilitate rather than burden care coordination efforts
- Quality improvement initiatives ensure continuous enhancement of integrated approaches while building organizational capacity for effective interdisciplinary collaboration

Chapter 18: Ready-to-Use Worksheets and Clinical Tools

The transition from theoretical knowledge to practical application requires concrete tools that group members can use independently while reinforcing therapeutic concepts learned during sessions. This collection of reproducible worksheets represents the bridge between group experiences and daily life implementation, providing structured formats that support skill development, self-monitoring, and therapeutic progress across diverse psychiatric conditions and cultural backgrounds.

Your role as a psychiatric nurse involves not only facilitating group discussions but also providing tangible resources that extend therapeutic benefits beyond formal session times. These worksheets serve as therapeutic interventions in themselves, offering structure and guidance that supports sustained recovery and skill generalization.

CBT Thought Records and Activity Logs

Cognitive Behavioral Therapy worksheets provide systematic frameworks for identifying thought patterns and tracking behavioral changes while building awareness of the connections between thoughts, feelings, and behaviors that drive psychiatric symptoms.

Worksheet CBT-1: Basic Thought Record

Instructions: Use this form whenever you notice a change in mood or feel upset. Complete each column to understand the connection between your thoughts and feelings.

Date/Time	Situation	Mood (1-10)	Automatic Thoughts	Evidence For	Evidence Against	Balanced Thought	New Mood (1-10)
	What happened?	How did you feel? Rate intensity	What went through your mind?	What supports this thought?	What contradicts this thought?	What's a more balanced view?	How do you feel now?

Case Example Application: Sarah, a 34-year-old teacher with depression, used this worksheet after feeling devastated when her supervisor suggested revisions to her lesson plan. Her automatic thought was "I'm a terrible teacher and everyone knows it." Through the evidence columns, she identified that her supervisor's feedback was actually constructive and that she had received positive evaluations previously. Her balanced thought became "Feedback helps me improve, and one suggestion doesn't define my teaching ability." Her mood improved from 8/10 (very upset) to 4/10 (mildly disappointed but manageable).

Worksheet CBT-2: Daily Activity Log

Instructions: Track your daily activities and mood to identify patterns. Rate mood and energy before and after each activity.

Time	Activity	Mood Before (1-10)	Energy Before (1-10)	Mood After (1-10)	Energy After (1-10)	Notes
7:00 AM						
9:00 AM						
11:00 AM						
1:00 PM						
3:00 PM						
5:00 PM						
7:00 PM						
9:00 PM						

Case Example Application: Marcus, a 28-year-old with depression, discovered through activity logging that his mood consistently dropped during unstructured afternoon hours when he isolated himself at home. His mood ratings showed a pattern: mornings at work (mood 6/10) dropped to afternoon isolation (mood 3/10) but improved with evening gym visits (mood 7/10). This data helped him schedule meaningful afternoon activities that prevented the daily mood decline.

Worksheet CBT-3: Behavioral Experiment Planning

Instructions: Use this worksheet to test negative predictions and gather evidence about feared situations.

Feared Situation: _____

Negative Prediction: _____

Anxiety Level (1-10): _____

Experiment Plan: What will you do? _____ When will you do it? _____ How will you measure success? _____

Safety Behaviors to Avoid: _____

Actual Outcome: What really happened? _____ How did you feel? _____ What did you learn? _____

Revised Prediction: _____

Worksheet CBT-4: Problem-Solving Worksheet

Instructions: Break down overwhelming problems into manageable steps using this structured approach.

Problem Description: _____

Goal: _____

Brainstorm Solutions:

1. _____
2. _____
3. _____
4. _____
5. _____

Evaluate Each Solution:

Solution	Pros	Cons	Feasibility (1-10)
1.			
2.			

Solution	Pros	Cons	Feasibility (1-10)
3.			

Selected Solution: _____

Action Steps:

1. _____
2. _____
3. _____

Timeline: _____

Obstacles and Solutions: _____

Worksheet CBT-5: Mood and Thought Monitoring

Instructions: Complete this weekly summary to track patterns in your thoughts and moods.

Week of: _____

Day	Lowest Mood (1-10)	Highest Mood (1-10)	Most Common Negative Thought	Helpful Coping Strategy Used	Notes
Monday					
Tuesday					
Wednesday					
Thursday					
Friday					
Saturday					
Sunday					

Weekly Reflection: What patterns do you notice? _____ What strategies were most helpful? _____ What would you like to focus on next week? _____

DBT Skills Practice Sheets

Dialectical Behavior Therapy worksheets provide structured practice opportunities for the four skills modules while helping group members track their skill use and effectiveness in daily situations.

Worksheet DBT-1: Mindfulness Skills Practice Log

Instructions: Record your daily mindfulness practice and track which techniques work best for you.

Date	Mindfulness Skill Used	Duration	Situation	Effectiveness (1-10)	Notes
	☐ Observe ☐ Describe ☐ Participate ☐ Non-judgmental ☐ One-mindfully ☐ Effectively				
	☐ Observe ☐ Describe ☐ Participate ☐ Non-judgmental ☐ One-mindfully ☐ Effectively				
	☐ Observe ☐ Describe ☐ Participate ☐ Non-judgmental ☐ One-mindfully ☐ Effectively				

Weekly Summary: Most helpful skill: _____ Most challenging situation: _____ Goal for next week: _____

Case Example Application: Jennifer, a 26-year-old with borderline personality disorder, used this log during a particularly stressful work week. She discovered that "observe" skills were most effective during interpersonal conflicts (effectiveness rating 8/10), while "participate" skills helped her stay focused during meetings (effectiveness rating 7/10). The log revealed that she used mindfulness skills more frequently on high-stress days, which corresponded with better emotional regulation.

Worksheet DBT-2: Distress Tolerance Skills Tracker

Instructions: Use this sheet to track crisis survival skills and their effectiveness during difficult moments.

Crisis Situation: _____

Distress Level Before (1-10): _____

Skills Used (check all that apply): ☐ TIPP (Temperature, Intense exercise, Paced breathing, Progressive muscle relaxation) ☐ Distraction (Activities, Contributing, Comparisons, Emotions, Push away, Thoughts, Sensations) ☐ Self-Soothing (Vision, Hearing, Smell, Taste, Touch) ☐ Improve the Moment (Imagery, Prayer, Relaxation, One thing at a time, Vacation, Encouragement, Meaning) ☐ Pros and Cons ☐ Radical Acceptance

Specific Techniques Used: _____

Distress Level After (1-10): _____

What worked best? _____

What would you do differently? _____

Case Example Application: David, a 32-year-old military veteran with PTSD, used this tracker during a flashback episode triggered by loud noises at a construction site. His initial distress level was 9/10. He used TIPP skills (cold water on face and paced breathing) and distraction techniques (counting objects in his environment). His distress level decreased to 4/10 within 20 minutes. The tracker helped him identify that combining TIPP with environmental grounding was most effective for his trauma responses.

Worksheet DBT-3: Emotion Regulation Worksheet

Instructions: Use this form to understand and work with difficult emotions.

Date: _____

Emotion: _____

Intensity (1-10): _____

Prompting Event: _____

Thoughts: _____

Body Sensations: _____

Action Urges: _____

What I Actually Did: _____

Consequences: Short-term: _____ Long-term: _____

Opposite Action (if emotion not justified): What would opposite action be? _____ Did I try it? _____ Result: _____

Self-Care Check: ☐ PLEASE skills maintained (Physical health, Eating, Avoiding substances, Sleep, Exercise) ☐ Mastery activity completed ☐ Pleasant activity completed

Worksheet DBT-4: Interpersonal Effectiveness Planning

Instructions: Prepare for difficult conversations using DEAR MAN, GIVE, and FAST skills.

Situation: _____

Relationship: _____

My Goal: _____

DEAR MAN Planning: Describe: _____ **E**xpress: _____ **A**ssert: _____ **R**einforce: _____ **M**indful: _____ **A**ppear confident: _____ **N**egotiate: _____

GIVE Planning: Gentle: _____ **I**nterested: _____ **V**alidate: _____ **E**asy manner: _____

FAST Planning: Fair: _____ **Apologies (no unnecessary):** _____ **Stick to values:** _____
Truthful: _____

Outcome: What happened? _____ How did I do with the skills? _____ What would I do differently? _____

Worksheet DBT-5: Daily Skills Review

Instructions: End each day by reflecting on your DBT skills practice.

Date: _____

Overall Mood (1-10): _____

Mindfulness: Did I practice mindful awareness today? ☐ Yes - How? _____ ☐ No - What got in the way? _____

Distress Tolerance: Did I handle distress skillfully? ☐ Yes - What skills did I use? _____ ☐ No - What could I try next time? _____

Emotion Regulation: Did I take care of my emotions? ☐ Yes - How? _____ ☐ No - What emotions were challenging? _____

Interpersonal Effectiveness: Were my relationships skillful? ☐ Yes - What went well? _____ ☐ No - What was difficult? _____

Tomorrow's Focus: _____

Mindfulness Exercise Scripts

Structured mindfulness scripts provide group members with guided practices they can use independently while building skills in present-moment awareness and acceptance.

Worksheet MIN-1: Progressive Muscle Relaxation Script

Instructions: Read through this script slowly, or have someone read it to you. Allow 15-20 minutes for the complete exercise.

Getting Started: Find a comfortable position, either sitting or lying down. Close your eyes or soften your gaze. Begin by taking three slow, deep breaths.

The Exercise: "Now we'll work through your body, tensing and then releasing each muscle group. Hold each tension for 5 seconds, then release and notice the contrast.

Feet and Legs: Point your toes and tense your feet... hold... and release. Feel the relaxation. Tighten your calf muscles... hold... and release. Tense your thigh muscles... hold... and release.

Abdomen and Back: Tighten your stomach muscles... hold... and release. Arch your back slightly... hold... and release.

Hands and Arms: Make fists and tense your hands... hold... and release. Tense your forearms... hold... and release. Tense your upper arms... hold... and release.

Shoulders and Neck: Raise your shoulders to your ears... hold... and release. Tense your neck muscles... hold... and release.

Face: Scrunch your forehead... hold... and release. Close your eyes tightly... hold... and release. Clench your jaw... hold... and release.

Finishing: Take three deep breaths and slowly open your eyes. Notice how your body feels now."

Practice Log: Date: _____ Duration: _____ Effectiveness (1-10): _____ Notes: _____

Worksheet MIN-2: Body Scan Meditation Guide

Instructions: Use this script for a 10-15 minute body scan practice.

Beginning: "Lie down comfortably and close your eyes. Take three deep breaths, allowing your body to settle.

The Scan: Start by bringing attention to the top of your head. Notice any sensations - warmth, coolness, tingling, or nothing at all. All sensations are welcome.

Move your attention to your forehead... your eyes... your cheeks... your jaw. Don't try to change anything, just notice.

Bring attention to your neck... your shoulders... your right arm... your left arm. Notice any tension or relaxation.

Focus on your chest... your breathing... your stomach... your back. Allow your breathing to be natural.

Move attention to your hips... your right leg... your left leg... your feet. Notice how your whole body feels supported.

Take a moment to sense your body as a whole... breathing... alive... present.

When ready, wiggle your fingers and toes, and slowly open your eyes."

Reflection Questions: What did you notice? _____
Where did you feel tension? _____ Where did you feel relaxed? _____ How do you feel now? _____

Case Example Application: Maria, a 38-year-old with anxiety disorder, used the body scan during her lunch breaks at work. She discovered that she held tension in her shoulders and jaw that she hadn't noticed before. Regular practice helped her recognize early signs of stress buildup, allowing her to use relaxation techniques before her anxiety escalated to panic levels.

Worksheet MIN-3: Breathing Exercise Instructions

Instructions: Choose one breathing technique based on your current needs.

4-7-8 Breathing (for anxiety):

1. Exhale completely
2. Inhale through nose for 4 counts
3. Hold breath for 7 counts
4. Exhale through mouth for 8 counts
5. Repeat 3-4 times

Box Breathing (for focus):

1. Inhale for 4 counts
2. Hold for 4 counts
3. Exhale for 4 counts
4. Hold for 4 counts
5. Repeat 5-10 times

Belly Breathing (for relaxation):

1. Place one hand on chest, one on belly
2. Breathe slowly through nose
3. Feel belly rise, chest stays still
4. Exhale slowly through mouth
5. Continue for 5-10 minutes

Practice Tracking:

Date	Technique Used	Duration	Before Stress (1-10)	After Stress (1-10)	Notes

Worksheet MIN-4: Mindful Walking Instructions

Instructions: Use this guide for 10-20 minute mindful walking practice.

Preparation: Choose a quiet path 10-20 steps long, either indoors or outdoors. Begin standing at one end.

The Practice:

1. **Standing:** Feel your feet on the ground. Notice your posture.
2. **Lifting:** Slowly lift your right foot. Notice the shift in weight.
3. **Moving:** Move your foot forward slowly. Feel the movement.
4. **Placing:** Place your foot down gently. Feel the contact.
5. **Repeat:** Continue with left foot. Walk very slowly.
6. **Turning:** At the path's end, turn around mindfully.
7. **Continue:** Walk back and forth for your chosen time.

When Mind Wanders:

- Simply notice where your mind went
- Gently return attention to walking
- No judgment needed

Reflection: What did you notice about walking? _____ How was this different from normal walking? _____ What thoughts or feelings came up? _____

Worksheet MIN-5: Five Senses Grounding Exercise

Instructions: Use this technique during anxiety, panic, or dissociation.

The 5-4-3-2-1 Technique:

5 Things You Can See: Look around and name 5 things you can see:

1. _____
2. _____
3. _____
4. _____
5. _____

4 Things You Can Touch: Notice 4 things you can feel:

1. _____
2. _____
3. _____
4. _____

3 Things You Can Hear: Listen for 3 sounds:

1. _____
2. _____
3. _____

2 Things You Can Smell: Notice 2 scents:

1. _____
2. _____

1 Thing You Can Taste: Notice 1 taste in your mouth:

1. _____

Check-In: How do you feel now? _____ Are you more present? _____

Case Example Application: Robert, a 34-year-old veteran with PTSD, used the 5-4-3-2-1 technique during flashback episodes. When triggered by loud noises that reminded him of combat, he would immediately begin naming things he could see around him. This grounding exercise helped him stay connected to present reality rather than being pulled into traumatic memories, reducing the intensity and duration of his flashback episodes.

Medication Tracking Forms

Systematic medication monitoring helps group members track therapeutic effects, side effects, and adherence patterns while building partnership with prescribers.

Worksheet MED-1: Daily Medication and Mood Log

Instructions: Complete this form daily to track your medications and how you're feeling.

Date: _____

Medication	Prescribed Dose	Time Taken	Dose Taken	Missed?	Notes
				☐ Yes ☐ No	
				☐ Yes ☐ No	
				☐ Yes ☐ No	
				☐ Yes ☐ No	

Daily Mood Ratings (1-10): Morning: _____ Afternoon: _____ Evening: _____

Side Effects Experienced: ☐ Nausea ☐ Dizziness ☐ Drowsiness ☐ Headache ☐ Dry mouth ☐ Weight changes ☐ Sleep problems ☐ Other: _____

Energy Level (1-10): _____

Sleep Quality (1-10): _____

Overall Day Rating (1-10): _____

Notes about your day: _____

Worksheet MED-2: Weekly Medication Review

Instructions: Complete this summary at the end of each week to track patterns.

Week of: _____

Medication Adherence: Percentage of doses taken as prescribed: _____ Most common reason for missed doses: _____

Mood Patterns: Highest mood this week: _____ Lowest mood this week: _____ Most common mood level: _____

Side Effects: Most bothersome side effect: _____ Side effects that improved: _____ New side effects: _____

Sleep and Energy: Average sleep quality (1-10): _____ Average energy level (1-10): _____

Questions for Prescriber:

1. _____
2. _____
3. _____

Goals for next week: _____

Case Example Application: Jennifer, a 28-year-old with bipolar disorder, used weekly medication reviews to track her lithium levels and mood stability. She noticed that her mood ratings were consistently lower on days when she took her medication late, and she experienced more side effects when she didn't maintain consistent timing. This data helped her prescriber adjust her dosing schedule and convinced Jennifer of the importance of medication consistency.

Worksheet MED-3: Side Effect Monitoring Form

Instructions: Use this form to track specific side effects and their impact on your daily life.

Medication: _____

Side Effect: _____

Date Started: _____

Date	Severity (1-10)	Duration	Impact on Daily Activities	Management Strategies Tried

Pattern Analysis: Does this side effect happen at specific times? _____ What makes it better? _____ What makes it worse? _____

Impact Assessment: How much does this affect your daily life? _____ How much does this affect your willingness to take medication? _____

Questions for Prescriber:

Worksheet MED-4: Medication Change Tracking

Instructions: Use this form when starting, stopping, or changing medications.

Medication Change: _____

Date Change Started: _____

Reason for Change: _____

Previous Medication/Dose: _____

New Medication/Dose: _____

Week 1 Observations: Mood changes: _____ Side effects: _____ Sleep changes: _____ Energy changes: _____

Week 2 Observations: Mood changes: _____ Side effects: _____ Sleep changes: _____ Energy changes: _____

Week 4 Observations: Overall improvement: _____ Ongoing concerns: _____ Questions for prescriber: _____

Worksheet MED-5: Medication Adherence Problem-Solving

Instructions: Use this worksheet when you're having trouble taking medications as prescribed.

Medication(s) I'm having trouble with: _____

Specific adherence problems (check all that apply): ☐ Forgetting to take medication ☐ Side effects are bothering me ☐ Don't think medication is helping ☐ Cost concerns ☐ Complicated schedule ☐ Don't like taking medication ☐ Other: _____

Most significant barrier: _____

Brainstorm Solutions:

1. _____
2. _____
3. _____
4. _____

Selected Solution to Try: _____

Implementation Plan: What will I do? _____ When will I start? _____ How will I track progress? _____

Support Needed: Who can help me? _____ What resources do I need? _____

Follow-up Plan: When will I review progress? _____ What would indicate success? _____

Safety Planning Templates

Structured safety planning provides group members with concrete strategies for managing suicidal thoughts, self-harm urges, or other crisis situations.

Worksheet SAFE-1: Personal Safety Plan

Instructions: Complete this plan with your therapist or trusted person. Keep copies in multiple places.

Warning Signs (thoughts, feelings, behaviors that indicate crisis):

1. _____
2. _____
3. _____
4. _____

Personal Coping Strategies (things I can do on my own):

1. _____
2. _____
3. _____
4. _____

People Who Can Help (name and phone number):

1. _____
2. _____
3. _____

Professional Contacts: Therapist: _____ Doctor: _____ Crisis Line: _____ Emergency Room: _____

Making My Environment Safe: Items to remove: _____
Safe storage plans: _____ People who can help: _____

Reasons to Live:

1. _____
2. _____
3. _____

Case Example Application: Michael, a 42-year-old construction worker with depression, developed his safety plan after experiencing suicidal thoughts following a job injury. His warning signs included isolating from family, drinking alcohol, and thinking "everyone would be better off without me." His coping strategies included calling his brother, going for walks, and listening to music. When he recognized his warning signs during a particularly difficult week, he used his plan to reach out to his brother and avoid alcohol, successfully managing the crisis without hospitalization.

Worksheet SAFE-2: Crisis Contact Card

Instructions: Keep this card with you at all times. Laminate for durability.

MY CRISIS CONTACT CARD

If I'm in crisis, I will call:

1. _____
2. _____
3. _____

24-Hour Crisis Lines: National Suicide Prevention Lifeline: 988 Crisis Text Line: Text HOME to 741741 Local Crisis Line: _____

Emergency Services: Emergency Room: _____ Police: 911 Paramedics: 911

My Safe Person: Name: _____ Phone: _____

My Therapist: Name: _____ Phone: _____

Quick Coping Reminders: • This feeling will pass • I have survived difficult times before • People care about me • Help is available

Worksheet SAFE-3: Self-Harm Alternative Strategies

Instructions: Use this worksheet to identify alternatives to self-harm when you feel the urge.

When I want to self-harm, I feel: _____

What I usually want from self-harm: ☐ To feel something ☐ To feel nothing ☐ To punish myself ☐ To release anger ☐ To communicate pain ☐ To feel in control ☐ Other: _____

Red Ice Cube Method (for pain sensation): Hold ice cubes in your hands or place on skin where you want to harm

Elastic Band Method (for physical sensation): Snap rubber band on wrist (safer than cutting)

Red Marker Method (for visual effect): Draw on skin with red washable marker

Exercise Alternatives:

- Run or walk vigorously
- Do jumping jacks
- Punch pillows
- Squeeze stress ball

Creative Alternatives:

- Draw your feelings
- Write angry letters (don't send)
- Play loud music
- Sculpt with clay

My Personal Alternatives:

1. _____

2. _____
3. _____
4. _____

After using alternatives: How do I feel? _____ What worked best? _____ What didn't work? _____

Worksheet SAFE-4: Emergency Action Plan

Instructions: Post this plan where you'll see it during crisis times.

STEP 1: RECOGNIZE THE CRISIS I know I'm in crisis when:

_____

STEP 2: IMMEDIATE SAFETY ☐ Remove means of harm ☐ Go to safe location ☐ Call safe person ☐ Use coping skills

STEP 3: GET HELP Call in this order: 1st: _____ 2nd: _____ 3rd: _____

STEP 4: PROFESSIONAL HELP If above doesn't help: ☐ Call crisis line: _____ ☐ Go to emergency room: _____ ☐ Call 911

STEP 5: FOLLOW-UP After crisis passes: ☐ Call therapist ☐ Review what happened ☐ Update safety plan ☐ Thank people who helped

Remember:

- Crisis feelings are temporary
- You have survived crises before
- Help is available 24/7
- You are worth saving

Worksheet SAFE-5: Recovery Wellness Plan

Instructions: Complete this plan to maintain your mental health and prevent crisis.

Daily Wellness Activities: Morning routine: _____
Exercise: _____ Nutrition: _____ Social connection: _____ Relaxation: _____

Weekly Wellness Activities: Social activities: _____
Creative activities: _____ Spiritual activities: _____ Nature activities: _____

Monthly Wellness Check: Medication review: _____
Therapy progress: _____ Goal setting: _____ Support system: _____

Warning Sign Monitoring: ☐ Sleep changes ☐ Appetite changes ☐ Mood changes ☐ Social withdrawal ☐ Neglecting self-care ☐ Substance use ☐ Hopeless thoughts ☐ Other: _____

When I notice warning signs, I will:

1. _____
2. _____
3. _____

Support System Check: Who supports my recovery? _____ How often do I connect with support? _____ What support do I need more of? _____

Case Example Application: Sarah, a 29-year-old new mother with postpartum depression, used her recovery wellness plan to maintain stability while caring for her infant. Her daily activities included a morning walk with the baby, calling her mother for support, and evening relaxation with her partner. When she noticed warning signs like increased crying and feeling overwhelmed, she activated her plan by asking for help with baby care and scheduling extra therapy sessions, preventing a crisis that could have required hospitalization.

Cultural Assessment Tools

Cultural assessment instruments help group facilitators understand how cultural background influences group participation while adapting interventions to honor diverse perspectives.

Worksheet CULT-1: Cultural Background Assessment

Instructions: Complete this form to help your healthcare team understand your cultural background and preferences.

Personal Information: Country of origin: _____
Languages spoken: _____ Primary language: _____ Generation in US (if applicable): _____ Religion/spirituality: _____

Family and Community: Family structure: _____
Important family roles: _____ Community connections: _____ Cultural celebrations: _____

Health and Healing Beliefs: What causes mental health problems in your culture? _____ Traditional healing practices: _____ Attitudes toward medication: _____ Attitudes toward therapy: _____

Communication Preferences: Direct vs. indirect communication: _____
Eye contact preferences: _____ Personal space preferences: _____ Touch/physical contact: _____

Group Participation: Comfort with sharing personal information: _____
Preference for individual vs. group activities: _____ Authority figures and respect: _____

Potential Barriers: Language barriers: _____
Transportation: _____ Childcare: _____ Work schedule: _____ Cultural conflicts: _____

Strengths and Resources: Cultural strengths: _____
Community resources: _____ Cultural coping strategies: _____

Worksheet CULT-2: Religious and Spiritual Assessment

Instructions: Share information about your spiritual beliefs and practices to help integrate them into your care.

Religious Affiliation: _____

Importance of Religion/Spirituality (1-10): _____

Religious Practices: ☐ Prayer ☐ Meditation ☐ Scripture reading ☐ Religious services ☐ Religious holidays ☐ Dietary restrictions ☐ Other: _____

Spiritual Beliefs About Mental Health: How does your faith view mental illness? _____ Are there religious conflicts with treatment? _____ What role should spirituality play in healing? _____

Religious Support System: Religious leader/pastor: _____
Religious community: _____ Spiritual mentor: _____

Prayer and Meditation: Do you pray/meditate? _____ What style? _____ When and where? _____

Religious Coping: How does faith help during difficult times? _____ What religious resources comfort you? _____ Are there spiritual practices you'd like to include in treatment? ___

Potential Conflicts: Are there treatments that conflict with beliefs? _____
Medical procedures with religious concerns? _____ Scheduling conflicts with religious observances? _____

Integration Requests: Would you like chaplain referral? _____ Prayer before sessions? _____ Religious materials available? _____

Case Example Application: Fatima, a 35-year-old Muslim woman with anxiety, used the religious assessment to communicate her needs for prayer time during group sessions and her concerns about male therapists. The assessment helped staff accommodate her five daily prayers and connect her with a female therapist, while incorporating Islamic concepts of patience and trust in Allah into her anxiety management strategies.

Worksheet CULT-3: Family Cultural Dynamics

Instructions: Describe your family's cultural patterns to help providers understand your context.

Family Structure: Who lives in your household? _____ Extended family involvement: _____ Family decision-making process: _____
_____

Gender Roles: Traditional male roles: _____ Traditional female roles: _____ How rigid are these roles? _____
_____

Authority and Respect: Who has authority in family decisions? _____ How is respect shown? _____ Rules about disagreeing with elders: _____

Communication Patterns: How does family handle conflict? _____ Is direct communication acceptable? _____ Who speaks for the family in medical situations? _____

Mental Health Attitudes: How does family view mental illness? _____ Stigma or shame associated with therapy? _____ Family support for treatment? _____

Cultural Stress Factors: Acculturation differences between generations: _____ Economic pressures: _____ Discrimination experiences: _____ Cultural identity conflicts: _____

Cultural Strengths: Family support systems: _____ Cultural wisdom and traditions: _____ Community connections: _____
_____

Treatment Preferences: Family involvement in treatment decisions: _____
Confidentiality concerns: _____ Cultural adaptations needed:
_____

Worksheet CULT-4: Acculturation Assessment

Instructions: This assessment helps understand your adaptation to mainstream culture and any related stress.

Background: Years in current country: _____ Age when immigrated (if applicable): _____ Reason for immigration:
_____

Language Use: Primary language at home: _____ Language with friends: _____ Language at work/school: _____ Language you think in: _____

Cultural Practices: Traditional foods eaten: _____
Traditional clothing worn: _____ Cultural holidays celebrated: _____ Traditional music/entertainment: _____

Social Connections: Friends from original culture (%): _____ Friends from mainstream culture (%): _____ Participate in cultural organizations: _____ Participate in mainstream organizations: _____

Values and Beliefs: Rate importance (1-10): Traditional cultural values: _____ Mainstream cultural values:
_____

Acculturation Stress: Conflicts between cultures: _____
Pressure to assimilate: _____ Loss of cultural identity: _____ Discrimination experiences: _____
_____

Intergenerational Differences: Differences with parents: _____ Differences with children: _____ Family conflicts about culture: _____
_____

Mental Health Impact: How does cultural stress affect mood? _____
Identity confusion: _____ Isolation feelings: _____

Worksheet CULT-5: Preferred Cultural Interventions

Instructions: Identify cultural elements you'd like included in your treatment.

Traditional Healing Preferences: ☐ Herbal remedies ☐ Spiritual cleansing ☐ Traditional healer consultation ☐ Religious rituals ☐ Community ceremony ☐ Family blessing ☐ Other: _____

Cultural Adaptation Requests: Communication style preferences: _____ Group composition preferences: _____
Treatment setting preferences: _____

Language Needs: ☐ Interpreter needed ☐ Bilingual materials ☐ Cultural concepts explained ☐ Traditional sayings/proverbs included

Family Involvement: Who should be included in treatment planning? _____ What information can be shared with family? _____ Cultural protocols for family meetings: _____

Religious Integration: ☐ Prayer included in sessions ☐ Religious texts referenced ☐ Chaplain consultation ☐ Religious holiday accommodation ☐ Other: _____

Community Resources: Cultural organizations to involve: _____
Traditional healers to consult: _____ Cultural mentors available: _____

Cultural Strengths to Build Upon: Cultural coping strategies: _____ Community support systems: _____ Traditional wisdom applicable: _____

Potential Barriers to Address: Cultural conflicts with treatment: _____ Stigma concerns in community: _____
Language or communication barriers: _____

Case Example Application: Juan, a 45-year-old Mexican immigrant with depression, used this worksheet to request that his treatment include traditional concepts of "nervios" and family involvement in his care. The assessment led to incorporating his understanding of depression as a spiritual imbalance, including his wife in treatment planning, and connecting him with a Spanish-speaking support group that honored his cultural values while providing evidence-based depression treatment.

Group Evaluation Forms

Systematic evaluation tools provide feedback about group effectiveness while identifying areas for improvement and building understanding of member experiences.

Worksheet EVAL-1: Session Feedback Form

Instructions: Complete this form after each group session to help improve the group experience.

Date: _____

Session Topic: _____

Overall Session Rating (1-10): _____

Content Evaluation: How relevant was today's topic to your needs? _____ How clearly was information presented? _____ How helpful were the activities? _____

Group Process: How comfortable did you feel participating? _____ How supportive were other group members? _____ How well did the facilitator manage the group? _____

Personal Benefit: What was most helpful about today's session? _____ What was least helpful? _____ What would you like more of? _____

Participation Level: How much did you participate today (1-10)? _____ What helped or hindered your participation? _____

Learning and Application: What did you learn today? _____ How will you apply this information? _____ What questions do you still have? _____

Suggestions: What would improve future sessions? _____ Topics you'd like to discuss: _____ Format changes you'd suggest: _____

Facilitator Feedback: What did the facilitator do well? _____ What could the facilitator improve? _____

Next Session: What are you looking forward to? _____ Any concerns about upcoming sessions? _____

Worksheet EVAL-2: Group Climate Assessment

Instructions: Rate your experience of the group atmosphere and relationships.

Group: _____

Week: _____

Rate each item (1 = Never, 5 = Always):

Engagement: Members are involved and participate actively: _____ Members seem interested in what others say: _____ Members give each other feedback: _____ There is sharing of personal material: _____

Avoidance: Members are distant and withdrawing: _____ Members seem bored or impatient: _____ Members avoid looking at each other: _____ There is little interaction between members: _____

Conflict: Members criticize and reject each other: _____ Members seem tense and anxious: _____ Members compete with each other: _____ There is friction and anger between members: _____

Support: Members care about each other: _____ Members trust each other: _____ Members understand each other: _____ Members accept each other: _____

Overall Group Atmosphere: How would you describe the group mood today? _____ Rate the overall group climate (1-10): _____

Safety and Trust: Do you feel safe in this group? _____ Can you be yourself in this group? _____ Do you trust other group members? _____

Case Example Application: The adolescent depression group used climate assessments to identify that conflict levels were high during weeks 4-6, with members criticizing each other's coping strategies. The facilitator used this data to address the competitive dynamics and implement group rules about supportive feedback. Subsequent assessments showed increased engagement and support scores, with members reporting feeling safer to share vulnerable experiences.

Worksheet EVAL-3: Therapeutic Factors Inventory

Instructions: Rate how much each factor has been helpful in your group experience.

Group: _____

Your time in group: _____

Rate each factor (1 = Not helpful, 5 = Extremely helpful):

Hope: Seeing others improve gives me hope: _____ The group gives me hope for my own recovery: _____

Universality: Learning I'm not alone in my problems: _____ Discovering others have similar experiences: _____

Information: Learning about my condition from the facilitator: _____ Getting advice and suggestions from members: _____

Altruism: Being able to help other group members: _____ Feeling useful and needed in the group: _____

Family Issues: Working through family-related problems: _____ Understanding my family patterns better: _____

Social Skills: Learning how to get along with people: _____ Practicing social skills in the group: _____

Imitation: Copying positive behaviors from others: _____ Learning new coping strategies from members: _____

Learning: Understanding my impact on others: _____ Getting feedback about my behavior: _____

Cohesion: Feeling accepted and belonging: _____ Caring about other group members: _____

Catharsis: Expressing feelings I usually keep inside: _____ Releasing pent-up emotions: _____

Existential: Finding meaning in my suffering: _____ Taking responsibility for my life: _____

Most Important Factors: Which three factors were most helpful for you?

1. _____
2. _____
3. _____

Worksheet EVAL-4: Individual Progress Review

Instructions: Complete this monthly review to track your personal progress in group.

Month: _____

Personal Goals Review: Goal 1: _____ Progress (1-10): _____ What helped progress? _____ What hindered progress? _____

Goal 2: _____ Progress (1-10): _____ What helped progress? _____ What hindered progress? _____

Goal 3: _____ Progress (1-10): _____ What helped progress? _____ What hindered progress? _____

Skill Development: New coping skills learned: _____ Skills you're using regularly: _____ Skills that need more practice: _____

Symptom Changes: Symptoms that have improved: _____
Symptoms that remain challenging: _____ Overall symptom management (1-10): _____

Relationship Changes: How have your relationships improved? _____
Group relationships that are helpful: _____ Social skills you've developed: _____

Behavioral Changes: Negative behaviors you've reduced: _____ Positive behaviors you've increased: _____ Habits you want to continue changing: _____

Quality of Life: Areas of life that have improved: _____ Daily functioning changes: _____ Overall life satisfaction (1-10): _____

Group Experience: How has the group helped you? _____ What aspects of group are most valuable? _____ What would you like to work on next? _____

Worksheet EVAL-5: Program Completion Survey

Instructions: Complete this comprehensive evaluation when you finish the group program.

Program: _____

Duration of participation: _____

Overall Program Rating (1-10): _____

Goal Achievement: Did you achieve your main goals? _____ Rate overall goal achievement (1-10): _____ What goals exceeded expectations? _____ What goals were harder than expected? _____

Program Components: Rate helpfulness (1-5): Educational content: _____ Group discussions: _____ Activities and exercises: _____ Handouts and worksheets: _____
Homework assignments: _____

Facilitator Evaluation: Knowledge and expertise: _____ Group management skills: _____ Supportiveness and empathy: _____ Availability and responsiveness: _____

Group Process: Group size: _____ Group composition: _____ Session length: _____ Program duration: _____

Benefits Received: Most significant benefit: _____
Unexpected benefits: _____ Skills you'll continue using: _____ Knowledge you'll apply: _____

Areas for Improvement: What would you change about the program? _____
Topics that need more time: _____ Additional resources needed: _____

Recommendation: Would you recommend this group? _____ Who would benefit most from this program? _____ What would you tell someone considering joining? _____

Follow-up Needs: What ongoing support do you need? _____ Interest in alumni or refresher groups? _____ Other services you'd like to access? _____

Case Example Application: At the completion of a 12-week CBT group for depression, completion surveys revealed that 85% of participants achieved their primary goals, with the most valued component being peer support (average rating 4.8/5). Members requested longer sessions for practicing skills and expressed interest in monthly alumni meetings. This feedback led to extending future groups from 90 to 120 minutes and establishing ongoing support groups for graduates.

Implementation Guidelines

These worksheets serve as therapeutic tools that extend group benefits into daily life while providing structured approaches to skill development and self-monitoring. Your role includes introducing worksheets appropriately, supporting completion, and integrating insights into ongoing group work.

Successful worksheet implementation requires attention to literacy levels, cultural considerations, and individual preferences while maintaining therapeutic value and promoting sustained engagement with recovery activities.

Essential Worksheet Applications

- CBT thought records and activity logs provide structured frameworks for cognitive restructuring and behavioral activation while building independent skill practice
- DBT skills practice sheets support daily application of mindfulness, distress tolerance, emotion regulation, and interpersonal effectiveness techniques
- Mindfulness exercise scripts offer guided practices for present-moment awareness while accommodating diverse comfort levels and trauma histories
- Medication tracking forms build partnership with prescribers while supporting informed treatment decisions and adherence improvement
- Safety planning templates provide concrete crisis management strategies while building confidence in survival skills and help-seeking abilities
- Cultural assessment tools ensure culturally responsive care while honoring diverse backgrounds and beliefs in group interventions
- Group evaluation forms support continuous quality improvement while capturing member experiences and program effectiveness data

Appendix A: Reproducible Worksheets and Handouts

The practical application of group therapy concepts requires concrete tools that group members can use independently while reinforcing learning and skill development beyond formal session times. These reproducible materials serve as bridges between group experiences and daily life application, providing structure and guidance that supports sustained therapeutic progress and skill generalization across various life situations.

Your collection of worksheets and handouts represents more than simple paperwork—these tools function as therapeutic interventions that extend your influence and support into group members' homes, workplaces, and communities where the real work of recovery happens between sessions.

CBT Thought Records and Activity Logs

Cognitive Behavioral Therapy worksheets provide structured frameworks for identifying and challenging negative thought patterns while tracking behavioral changes that support mental health recovery and skill development.

Basic Thought Record captures the fundamental CBT model with columns for situation, mood, automatic thoughts, evidence for and against thoughts, balanced thoughts, and new mood ratings. This simple format helps group members practice cognitive restructuring independently while building awareness of thought-feeling-behavior connections.

Daily Thought Log encourages regular practice of thought monitoring while providing space for recording multiple thinking episodes throughout each day. This extended format builds habits of self-observation while increasing awareness of thinking patterns that occur outside therapeutic settings.

Behavioral Experiment Worksheet guides members through testing negative predictions while recording actual outcomes compared to feared consequences. This tool builds confidence in facing anxiety-provoking situations while gathering evidence that challenges catastrophic thinking patterns.

Activity Scheduling Form helps members plan pleasant and meaningful activities while tracking mood changes associated with different types of engagement. This behavioral activation tool counters depression and withdrawal while building momentum for increased life participation.

Problem-Solving Worksheet provides step-by-step guidance for addressing life challenges while breaking overwhelming situations into manageable components. This structured approach builds confidence in members' capacity for handling difficulties independently.

Case Example: Thought Record Implementation in Anxiety Group

Our anxiety management group discovered that providing structured thought record templates significantly improved members' ability to practice cognitive restructuring techniques between sessions while building skills for managing anxiety symptoms in real-world situations.

Jennifer, a 28-year-old teacher with social anxiety, initially struggled to identify her automatic thoughts during anxiety episodes, finding herself overwhelmed by physical symptoms without awareness of the cognitive processes that triggered her panic responses.

The **situation column** helped Jennifer identify specific triggers for her anxiety while building awareness that her symptoms had identifiable causes rather than appearing randomly or without reason.

Mood rating scales (1-10) provided objective measures of her emotional intensity while helping her track improvements and recognize that emotions naturally fluctuate rather than remaining constant.

Automatic thought identification became easier with practice as Jennifer learned to pause during anxiety episodes and ask herself "What am I thinking right now?" rather than focusing solely on physical symptoms.

Evidence columns helped Jennifer evaluate the accuracy of her anxiety-provoking thoughts while building skills in realistic thinking rather than accepting anxious predictions without question.

Balanced thinking development showed Jennifer that she could acknowledge genuine concerns while avoiding catastrophic interpretations that increased her anxiety unnecessarily.

Jennifer's consistent use of thought records led to significant improvements in her anxiety management while building confidence in her ability to handle social situations that had previously felt overwhelming.

DBT Skills Practice Sheets

Dialectical Behavior Therapy worksheets provide structured practice opportunities for the four skills modules while helping group members track their skill use and effectiveness in daily life situations.

Mindfulness Practice Log records daily mindfulness activities while tracking duration, techniques used, and effectiveness ratings. This log builds habits of mindful awareness while providing data about which techniques work best for individual group members.

Distress Tolerance Skills Tracker documents use of crisis survival skills while recording situations that triggered skill use and outcomes achieved. This tracking builds confidence in members' capacity for surviving emotional crises without making situations worse.

Emotion Regulation Worksheet guides members through identifying emotions, understanding their functions, and choosing appropriate responses while building emotional intelligence and regulation skills.

Interpersonal Effectiveness Planning Sheet helps members prepare for difficult conversations while using DEAR MAN, GIVE, and FAST skills to achieve their goals while maintaining relationships and self-respect.

Daily Skills Practice Card provides quick reference for DBT skills while encouraging consistent practice and building familiarity with skill options during emotionally intense situations.

Mindfulness Exercise Scripts

Structured mindfulness scripts provide group members with guided practices they can use independently while building skills in present-moment awareness and acceptance that support emotional regulation and stress reduction.

Progressive Muscle Relaxation Script guides members through systematic tensing and releasing of muscle groups while building awareness of the connection between physical tension and emotional stress.

Guided Imagery Exercises provide detailed descriptions of peaceful settings while engaging multiple senses to create calming mental experiences that can be accessed during stressful situations.

Body Scan Instructions lead members through systematic attention to physical sensations while building mindful awareness of bodily experiences without judgment or attempts to change them.

Breathing Exercise Guidelines offer various breathing techniques including diaphragmatic breathing, counted breathing, and breathing with visualization while providing tools for immediate anxiety and stress management.

Walking Meditation Directions adapt mindfulness practice for movement while providing opportunities for practice that doesn't require sitting still or closing eyes, making mindfulness accessible for individuals with trauma histories or attention difficulties.

Case Example: Mindfulness Scripts for PTSD Group

Our trauma recovery group required carefully adapted mindfulness scripts that maintained safety while building present-moment awareness skills for individuals whose hypervigilance and dissociation made traditional meditation approaches potentially triggering.

Robert, a 34-year-old military veteran with combat PTSD, found that standard mindfulness exercises increased his anxiety rather than providing the calming effects other group members experienced.

Eyes-open adaptations allowed Robert to maintain visual connection with his environment while practicing mindfulness, reducing triggers associated with closing eyes and becoming vulnerable to surprise.

Grounding-focused scripts helped Robert connect with his physical environment while using sensory awareness to interrupt dissociative episodes and maintain present-moment orientation.

Choice-emphasis modifications gave Robert control over his participation level while respecting his need for autonomy and safety during vulnerable mindfulness practice.

Shortened versions accommodated Robert's limited attention span while providing meaningful mindfulness experiences that didn't overwhelm his capacity for present-moment awareness.

Movement integration combined mindfulness with gentle physical activity while addressing Robert's need for vigilance and readiness for action that sitting meditation couldn't accommodate.

Robert's successful adaptation of mindfulness practices demonstrated the importance of flexible approaches while building his confidence in using these tools for managing PTSD symptoms in daily life.

Medication Tracking Forms

Systematic medication monitoring provides group members with tools for tracking therapeutic effects, side effects, and adherence patterns while building partnership with prescribers and informed participation in treatment decisions.

Daily Medication Log records medication times, doses taken, side effects experienced, and mood or symptom changes while providing data for medication adjustments and adherence improvement strategies.

Side Effect Monitoring Form tracks specific adverse effects including onset timing, severity ratings, and impact on daily functioning while helping members communicate effectively with prescribers about medication experiences.

Mood and Medication Tracker combines medication adherence with mood ratings while building awareness of the connection between consistent medication use and symptom improvement.

Medication Schedule Template provides weekly planning grids while helping members organize complex medication regimens and coordinate timing with daily activities and meals.

Questions for Prescriber Worksheet helps members prepare for medication appointments while ensuring that important concerns and observations are communicated effectively during brief clinical encounters.

Safety Planning Templates

Structured safety planning provides group members with concrete strategies for managing suicidal thoughts, self-harm urges, or other crisis situations while building confidence in their capacity for survival and help-seeking.

Crisis Survival Plan identifies warning signs, coping strategies, support contacts, and emergency resources while providing step-by-step guidance for managing acute suicidal thoughts or self-harm urges.

Personal Safety Network maps formal and informal support resources while building understanding of help options available during different types of crises and emotional emergencies.

Coping Strategy Menu lists multiple techniques for managing difficult emotions while providing options that accommodate different situations, energy levels, and personal preferences.

Environmental Safety Checklist guides members through removing or securing potentially dangerous items while creating safer living environments that support recovery rather than increasing risk.

Help-Seeking Protocol provides specific steps for accessing professional help while overcoming barriers such as shame, cost concerns, or previous negative experiences with mental health services.

Case Example: Safety Planning for Borderline Personality Group

Our borderline personality disorder skills group required individualized safety planning approaches that addressed the complex self-harm behaviors and suicidal thoughts common in this population while building skills for crisis management and emotional regulation.

Maria, a 26-year-old with BPD, had a history of self-cutting and multiple suicide attempts, requiring a safety plan that addressed both impulsive self-harm and planned suicide attempts.

Warning sign identification helped Maria recognize early signs of emotional dysregulation while building awareness that could support early intervention before reaching crisis levels.

Coping skills hierarchy organized Maria's strategies from immediate crisis interventions to longer-term emotion regulation while providing multiple options for different situations and emotional intensities.

Support network mapping identified people Maria could contact during different types of crises while building understanding of appropriate support for various emotional needs and situations.

Means restriction planning addressed Maria's access to self-harm tools while developing strategies for creating safer environments during high-risk periods.

Professional resource coordination connected Maria's safety plan with her treatment team while ensuring that all providers understood her crisis management strategies and support needs.

Maria's safety plan implementation contributed to a significant reduction in both self-harm episodes and emergency department visits while building her confidence in managing emotional crises independently.

Cultural Assessment Tools

Cultural assessment instruments help group facilitators understand how cultural background influences group participation while adapting interventions to honor diverse perspectives and values.

Cultural Background Questionnaire explores ethnicity, language preferences, immigration history, and acculturation levels while building understanding of cultural factors that might affect group engagement and therapeutic relationships.

Religious and Spiritual Assessment examines faith traditions, spiritual practices, and beliefs about mental illness while identifying religious resources that could support recovery efforts.

Family and Community Mapping identifies cultural supports and potential conflicts while building understanding of collective versus individual decision-making patterns that might influence treatment engagement.

Communication Style Inventory assesses preferences for direct versus indirect communication while adapting group facilitation approaches to honor diverse cultural communication patterns.

Healing Tradition Survey explores traditional healing practices and cultural approaches to mental health while building bridges between cultural wisdom and evidence-based treatments.

Group Evaluation Forms

Systematic evaluation tools provide feedback about group effectiveness while identifying areas for improvement and building understanding of member experiences and satisfaction.

Session Rating Scales capture immediate feedback about individual sessions while tracking changes in member satisfaction and engagement over time.

Group Climate Assessment measures member perceptions of safety, support, and therapeutic benefit while identifying group dynamics that either support or hinder therapeutic progress.

Therapeutic Factors Inventory evaluates which aspects of group experience members find most helpful while guiding facilitation adjustments and intervention modifications.

Progress Tracking Forms document individual member advancement toward personal goals while providing data for treatment planning and outcome evaluation.

Program Feedback Survey captures overall impressions of group experiences while identifying strengths and areas for improvement in program design and implementation.

Creating Effective Worksheets

Successful therapeutic worksheets require careful design that balances structure with flexibility while accommodating diverse learning styles and cognitive abilities.

Clear instructions use simple language and step-by-step guidance while avoiding jargon or complex directions that might confuse or intimidate group members.

Adequate space provides room for thoughtful responses while avoiding overwhelming blank spaces that might feel intimidating for members with writing difficulties or processing challenges.

Visual appeal uses fonts, spacing, and design elements that feel professional yet approachable while creating materials that members feel proud to use and share.

Cultural sensitivity considers how language, examples, and concepts translate across diverse populations while ensuring that materials feel relevant and respectful to all group members.

Flexibility options allow for different types of responses while accommodating varying literacy levels, physical abilities, and personal preferences for self-expression.

Distribution and Follow-up

Effective use of worksheets requires systematic approaches to distribution, completion tracking, and follow-up that integrate these tools meaningfully into group processes.

Introduction timing presents new worksheets at appropriate moments while building understanding of their purpose and connection to group goals and individual recovery objectives.

Completion support provides assistance for members who struggle with written materials while ensuring that everyone can participate regardless of literacy levels or learning differences.

Review processes dedicate group time to discussing worksheet experiences while building learning from both successful applications and implementation challenges.

Modification encouragement supports members in adapting worksheets to meet their individual needs while maintaining therapeutic value and promoting personalized recovery approaches.

Progress integration connects worksheet insights to broader treatment planning while ensuring that independent work contributes meaningfully to overall therapeutic progress and goal achievement.

Resource Development

The creation and refinement of therapeutic worksheets represents ongoing process that benefits from member feedback, facilitator experience, and evolving understanding of effective group interventions.

Successful worksheet development requires attention to member needs, cultural considerations, and practical implementation challenges while building resources that truly support therapeutic goals rather than creating busy work that feels disconnected from recovery objectives.

Essential Resource Components

- CBT thought records and activity logs provide structured frameworks for cognitive restructuring and behavioral activation while building independent skill practice opportunities
- DBT skills practice sheets support daily application of mindfulness, distress tolerance, emotion regulation, and interpersonal effectiveness techniques
- Mindfulness exercise scripts offer guided practices for present-moment awareness while accommodating trauma histories and diverse comfort levels
- Medication tracking forms build partnership with prescribers while supporting informed treatment decisions and adherence improvement
- Safety planning templates provide concrete crisis management strategies while building confidence in survival skills and help-seeking abilities
- Cultural assessment tools and group evaluation forms ensure culturally responsive care while supporting continuous program improvement and member satisfaction

Appendix B: Assessment Tools and Outcome Measures

The systematic measurement of therapeutic progress requires validated instruments that capture both symptom changes and functional improvements while providing objective data that supports evidence-based practice and demonstrates the effectiveness of group interventions. These assessment tools serve as both clinical guides and accountability measures that ensure your group work produces measurable benefits for participants.

Your selection and use of assessment instruments reflects your commitment to professional excellence while providing the data necessary for treatment planning, progress monitoring, and outcome evaluation that supports both individual care and program development.

Beck Depression Inventory (BDI-II)

The Beck Depression Inventory remains one of the most widely used and validated measures of depressive symptoms, providing reliable assessment that supports both clinical decision-making and research activities (33). This 21-item self-report questionnaire captures the cognitive, emotional, and physical symptoms of depression while offering standardized scoring that allows for comparison across individuals and treatment settings.

Symptom domains assessed include sadness, pessimism, guilt, concentration difficulties, sleep disturbances, and appetite changes while providing complete picture of depression presentation rather than focusing on single symptoms or narrow aspects of mood disorders.

Severity scoring ranges from minimal depression (0-13) through mild (14-19), moderate (20-28), and severe depression (29-63) while providing clear guidelines for treatment intensity and urgency that support clinical decision-making.

Change sensitivity allows detection of improvement over time while providing objective measures of treatment response that complement clinical observations and subjective reports from group members.

Treatment planning applications use BDI-II scores to guide intervention selection while monitoring progress toward recovery goals and identifying individuals who may need additional support or modified treatment approaches.

Group therapy adaptations involve administering the BDI-II before, during, and after group participation while tracking both individual member progress and overall group effectiveness in addressing depressive symptoms.

GAD-7 Anxiety Scale

The Generalized Anxiety Disorder 7-item scale provides brief yet effective screening and monitoring for anxiety symptoms while offering practical assessment that can be completed quickly without burdening group members or consuming excessive session time.

Core anxiety symptoms measured include excessive worry, restlessness, fatigue, concentration difficulties, irritability, muscle tension, and sleep problems while capturing the essential features of anxiety disorders.

Scoring interpretation uses cutoff points of 5, 10, and 15 for mild, moderate, and severe anxiety respectively while providing clear guidelines for treatment recommendations and intensity decisions.

Weekly administration tracks anxiety changes over time while providing data for adjusting group interventions and identifying members who may need additional individual support or medication evaluation.

Treatment response monitoring documents improvement in anxiety symptoms while providing objective evidence of group therapy effectiveness for both clinical and administrative purposes.

Risk assessment support identifies individuals with severe anxiety who may need immediate attention while ensuring that high-risk members receive appropriate care and monitoring.

Patient Health Questionnaire (PHQ-9)

The PHQ-9 provides standardized assessment of depression symptoms while offering practical screening tool that supports both diagnosis and treatment monitoring in various healthcare settings (34). This nine-item questionnaire directly corresponds to DSM-5 criteria for major depression while providing user-friendly format that group members can complete independently.

Diagnostic alignment with DSM-5 criteria supports accurate assessment while ensuring that symptom evaluation matches current diagnostic standards and clinical practice guidelines.

Functional impairment measurement includes questions about how symptoms affect work, relationships, and daily activities while providing data about real-world impact beyond symptom severity scores.

Suicide screening incorporates questions about death wishes and self-harm thoughts while providing essential safety information that requires immediate clinical attention and follow-up.

Treatment tracking through repeated administration documents symptom changes while providing evidence for treatment effectiveness and areas needing additional intervention focus.

Quality improvement applications use PHQ-9 data for program evaluation while demonstrating group therapy outcomes to administrators and funding sources who require objective outcome measures.

Case Example: Integrating Multiple Assessment Tools

Our mixed diagnostic group utilized multiple assessment instruments to capture the complex presentations of twelve group members with various psychiatric conditions while building understanding of treatment effectiveness across different symptom domains and functional areas.

Sarah, a 35-year-old with comorbid depression and anxiety, demonstrated the value of multiple assessments in tracking her complex presentation and treatment response patterns.

Baseline assessments revealed moderate depression (BDI-II score of 24) and severe anxiety (GAD-7 score of 16) while providing clear targets for group intervention and individual treatment planning.

Weekly monitoring showed that Sarah's anxiety improved more rapidly than her depression, with GAD-7 scores decreasing to moderate levels by week four while BDI-II scores remained in the moderate range until week eight.

Functional measures indicated that work performance improved before mood symptoms while demonstrating that group therapy benefits extended beyond symptom reduction to include practical life improvements.

Treatment adjustments used assessment data to modify group activities while increasing focus on behavioral activation techniques when depression scores plateaued despite continued anxiety improvement.

Outcome documentation showed significant improvements in both depression and anxiety by group completion while providing evidence for treatment effectiveness that supported continued funding and program expansion.

Sarah's multi-domain assessment demonstrated the value of using various instruments while building understanding of how different symptoms respond to group interventions at different rates and through different mechanisms.

Health of the Nation Outcome Scales (HoNOS)

The HoNOS provides comprehensive assessment of mental health and social functioning while offering standardized measurement that captures the broader impact of psychiatric conditions beyond symptom severity (35). This 12-item scale addresses behavior, impairment, symptoms, and social functioning while providing holistic evaluation appropriate for complex psychiatric presentations.

Behavioral assessment measures aggression, self-harm, and substance use while providing safety information that guides group participation decisions and crisis planning.

Functional evaluation examines cognitive problems, physical illness, and hallucinations while building understanding of how various impairments affect group participation and treatment response.

Social functioning assessment covers relationships, daily living skills, and housing while measuring areas that group therapy specifically targets through peer support and skill development.

Change measurement tracks improvements across multiple domains while providing evidence for broad therapeutic benefits that extend beyond symptom reduction to include quality of life improvements.

Program evaluation uses HoNOS data to demonstrate comprehensive treatment outcomes while supporting funding requests and quality improvement initiatives that require evidence of effectiveness.

Group Cohesion Scales

Group cohesion measurement captures the therapeutic relationships and group dynamics that drive healing processes while providing data about group functioning that guides facilitation decisions and program improvements.

Therapeutic climate assessment measures group warmth, support, and acceptance while identifying groups that may need intervention to improve therapeutic relationships and member engagement.

Conflict evaluation documents tension and disagreement patterns while building understanding of group dynamics that might interfere with therapeutic progress and member satisfaction.

Engagement measurement tracks member participation and investment while identifying individuals who may need additional support or modified approaches to increase their group involvement.

Leadership assessment evaluates member perceptions of facilitator effectiveness while providing feedback for professional development and group management improvement.

Outcome correlation connects cohesion scores with treatment results while building understanding of group factors that predict successful therapeutic outcomes.

Session Rating Scales

Immediate feedback about individual session experiences provides real-time data for adjusting group activities while ensuring that interventions meet member needs and maintain therapeutic engagement.

Session satisfaction captures member reactions to specific activities while identifying interventions that feel most helpful and engaging for different individuals and group compositions.

Relevance evaluation measures how well session content addresses member concerns while ensuring that group activities connect meaningfully to individual recovery goals and treatment needs.

Facilitator feedback provides information about leadership effectiveness while supporting professional development and improvement in group management skills.

Participation comfort assesses how safe and supported members feel while identifying barriers to engagement that might require attention or modification.

Learning assessment evaluates knowledge gained and skills developed while ensuring that educational components achieve their intended objectives and support therapeutic progress.

Treatment Satisfaction Surveys

Overall program evaluation captures member perspectives on group therapy experiences while providing data for quality improvement and program development activities.

Global satisfaction measures overall happiness with group participation while identifying programs that successfully meet member needs and expectations for treatment.

Specific component evaluation examines different aspects of group programming while building understanding of which elements contribute most to member satisfaction and therapeutic benefit.

Recommendation likelihood assesses whether members would suggest group therapy to others while providing data about program quality and member loyalty.

Improvement suggestions gather specific feedback about program modifications while engaging members as partners in quality improvement and program development efforts.

Value perception measures whether members believe group therapy was worth their time and effort while providing data about treatment acceptability and member investment.

Case Example: Comprehensive Outcome Measurement

Our dual diagnosis program implemented extensive outcome measurement to demonstrate effectiveness while building understanding of which interventions produced the best results for individuals with co-occurring mental health and substance use disorders.

Michael, a 29-year-old with bipolar disorder and alcohol use disorder, participated in comprehensive assessment that tracked multiple outcome domains throughout his twelve-week group participation.

Baseline measurements established his starting point across symptom severity, functional status, and treatment engagement while providing targets for intervention and progress monitoring.

Weekly assessments tracked symptom changes in both mental health and substance use domains while building understanding of how improvements in one area affected the other condition.

Functional outcomes measured work performance, relationship quality, and daily living skills while documenting improvements that extended beyond symptom reduction to include quality of life gains.

Treatment engagement monitored group attendance, homework completion, and active participation while identifying factors that supported or hindered his involvement in treatment activities.

Long-term follow-up continued assessment for six months after group completion while building understanding of sustained benefits and areas needing ongoing support or intervention.

Michael's outcome data demonstrated significant improvements across all measured domains while providing evidence for integrated treatment effectiveness that supported program continuation and expansion.

Selecting Appropriate Measures

Effective outcome measurement requires careful selection of instruments that match program goals while balancing assessment burden with data quality and clinical utility.

Population considerations ensure that chosen measures are appropriate for specific demographics while accounting for cultural factors, literacy levels, and cognitive abilities that might affect assessment validity.

Symptom specificity matches instruments to primary treatment targets while ensuring that assessments capture the specific changes that group interventions are designed to produce.

Time efficiency balances measurement quality with practical constraints while selecting instruments that provide valuable data without overwhelming group members or consuming excessive session time.

Psychometric quality prioritizes validated instruments with established reliability and validity while ensuring that assessment data meets professional standards for clinical and research applications.

Clinical utility emphasizes measures that inform treatment decisions while selecting instruments that provide actionable information for ongoing care planning and intervention modification.

Data Management and Analysis

Systematic approaches to outcome data ensure that assessment information supports both clinical care and program evaluation while maintaining confidentiality and meeting regulatory requirements.

Data collection protocols establish consistent procedures while ensuring that assessments are administered properly and results are recorded accurately and completely.

Confidentiality protection safeguards member privacy while allowing for appropriate data sharing that supports treatment planning and quality improvement activities.

Statistical analysis examines outcome patterns while identifying trends and relationships that inform program development and intervention refinement.

Report generation communicates findings to stakeholders while providing evidence for program effectiveness and areas needing improvement or additional resources.

Quality assurance monitors data integrity while ensuring that assessment information accurately represents member experiences and treatment outcomes.

Building Assessment Culture

Successful outcome measurement requires organizational commitment while building culture that values data-driven decision-making and continuous improvement in group therapy programming.

Creating assessment systems that support rather than burden clinical care requires careful planning and implementation while ensuring that measurement activities contribute meaningfully to therapeutic goals rather than feeling like administrative requirements.

Measurement Foundations

- Beck Depression Inventory and PHQ-9 provide validated depression assessment while supporting treatment planning and progress monitoring for mood disorder groups
- GAD-7 Anxiety Scale offers brief yet effective anxiety measurement while tracking treatment response and identifying high-risk individuals
- HoNOS captures comprehensive functioning while measuring broad therapeutic benefits that extend beyond symptom reduction
- Group cohesion scales assess therapeutic relationships while providing data about group dynamics that drive healing processes
- Session rating scales and treatment satisfaction surveys provide immediate feedback while supporting continuous quality improvement
- Multiple assessment domains ensure complete outcome measurement while demonstrating group therapy effectiveness across various therapeutic targets

Appendix C: Documentation Templates

The systematic documentation of group therapy services requires standardized templates that capture both individual member progress and group-level dynamics while meeting regulatory requirements and supporting quality improvement initiatives. These templates serve as both clinical tools and legal records that protect both patients and providers while demonstrating the value and effectiveness of group interventions.

Your documentation practices reflect your professional competence while providing the detailed records necessary for continuity of care, regulatory compliance, and evidence-based practice development that supports the advancement of group therapy as a legitimate and effective treatment modality.

Group Progress Note Formats

Structured progress note templates ensure consistent documentation while capturing the essential elements of group therapy sessions in formats that meet both clinical and regulatory requirements.

SOAP Format Adaptation modifies the traditional Subjective, Objective, Assessment, and Plan structure for group settings while maintaining familiar documentation patterns that integrate seamlessly with other healthcare records.

The **Subjective section** captures group members' verbal reports about their experiences, concerns, and progress while documenting relevant disclosures and self-assessments that inform treatment planning and risk evaluation.

Objective observations record facilitator observations of group dynamics, individual behaviors, participation patterns, and therapeutic responses while providing factual information that supports clinical assessment and intervention decisions.

Assessment components synthesize group session information while providing clinical judgments about individual progress, group functioning, and therapeutic effectiveness that guide ongoing treatment planning.

Plan elements outline follow-up activities, homework assignments, and future session goals while ensuring continuity between sessions and coordination with other treatment providers and interventions.

DAP Format Application uses Data, Assessment, and Plan structure while providing alternative documentation approach that some practitioners find more suitable for group therapy settings and interdisciplinary communication.

Case Example: SOAP Documentation Implementation

Our intensive outpatient program required detailed group therapy documentation that met both accreditation standards and insurance requirements while supporting clinical care and treatment planning for diverse patient populations.

The **Subjective section** for a depression group session documented member reports including "I felt more hopeful after hearing how others overcame similar problems" and "I'm still struggling with getting out of bed, but the group gives me something to look forward to."

Objective observations recorded specific behaviors such as "Client A arrived 10 minutes late, made eye contact with other members, participated actively in check-in, and offered support to Client B during crisis disclosure" while providing factual information for clinical assessment.

Assessment statements synthesized session information: "Group demonstrated increasing cohesion with members spontaneously offering support to each other. Client A showed improved engagement compared to previous sessions, while Client B's crisis disclosure was handled appropriately by both facilitator and group members."

Plan documentation outlined specific follow-up activities: "Continue current group format, provide individual check-in with Client B before next session, assign behavioral activation homework to all members, and review group rules about crisis disclosures."

This structured approach ensured consistent documentation while capturing both individual and group-level information necessary for treatment planning and regulatory compliance.

Attendance Tracking Sheets

Systematic attendance documentation provides data for treatment planning while meeting insurance requirements and supporting program evaluation activities that demonstrate group therapy utilization and effectiveness.

Member identification includes sufficient information for record-keeping while protecting confidentiality and ensuring accurate tracking of individual participation patterns over time.

Session dates and times provide complete scheduling information while documenting program compliance with planned treatment schedules and allowing for make-up session planning.

Attendance status records present, absent, late arrival, or early departure while building understanding of participation patterns that might affect treatment outcomes and engagement.

Reason codes document excused absences, medical conflicts, or other factors affecting attendance while providing data for identifying barriers to participation that might require intervention.

Cumulative tracking calculates attendance percentages while providing data for treatment planning and insurance reporting that requires documentation of minimum participation levels.

Behavioral Observation Forms

Structured observation templates ensure consistent recording of therapeutically relevant behaviors while providing objective data that supports treatment planning and outcome evaluation.

Participation level measures verbal contributions, nonverbal engagement, and interaction with other members while tracking changes in group involvement over time that indicate therapeutic progress.

Mood presentation documents observable signs of depression, anxiety, agitation, or other emotional states while providing information for safety assessment and treatment planning.

Social interaction records peer relationships, conflict patterns, and supportive behaviors while building understanding of interpersonal functioning that group therapy specifically addresses.

Coping skill demonstration tracks use of therapeutic techniques during group sessions while providing evidence of skill acquisition and application that supports treatment effectiveness.

Crisis indicators documents warning signs of emotional distress or risk behaviors while ensuring appropriate follow-up and safety planning for vulnerable group members.

Incident Report Templates

Standardized incident documentation ensures appropriate response to group crises while meeting legal requirements and supporting quality improvement activities that prevent future occurrences.

Incident description provides factual account of events while avoiding subjective interpretations or blame that might compromise legal protection or therapeutic relationships.

Individuals involved identifies all parties affected while protecting confidentiality and ensuring appropriate follow-up care for everyone impacted by the incident.

Timeline documentation records sequence of events while providing detailed chronology that supports investigation and quality improvement activities.

Intervention actions describes immediate responses and follow-up care while documenting appropriate clinical decision-making and crisis management procedures.

Outcome assessment evaluates incident resolution while identifying lessons learned and system improvements that could prevent similar occurrences in future.

Case Example: Incident Documentation for Group Crisis

Our borderline personality disorder group experienced a crisis when one member disclosed active suicidal ideation during a routine session, requiring immediate intervention and careful documentation.

Incident description recorded: "At 10:45 AM during group check-in, Client X stated 'I don't think I can make it through another day' and disclosed specific suicide plan involving medication overdose. Client appeared tearful and agitated."

Timeline documentation provided detailed sequence: "10:45 - Crisis disclosure made, 10:46 - Group facilitator implemented crisis protocol, 10:50 - Other group members moved to adjacent room with co-facilitator, 10:55 - Individual assessment begun with Client X."

Intervention actions described immediate responses: "Crisis assessment completed using Columbia Suicide Severity Rating Scale, family contact made, psychiatrist consulted, safety plan developed, and emergency department transport arranged."

Follow-up planning documented ongoing care: "Client X will be assessed by emergency psychiatrist, group will process incident at next session, individual members will receive check-in calls, and crisis protocols will be reviewed with staff."

This documentation provided complete record while protecting all parties and supporting quality improvement activities.

Outcome Summary Reports

Periodic summary documentation synthesizes individual progress while providing data for treatment planning, insurance reporting, and program evaluation activities.

Progress toward goals measures advancement on individual treatment objectives while providing evidence of therapeutic benefit and areas needing continued attention or intervention modification.

Skill development documents acquisition of coping strategies while providing evidence of learning and behavioral change that supports treatment effectiveness and member empowerment.

Functional improvements tracks changes in daily living abilities while measuring real-world benefits that extend beyond symptom reduction to include quality of life gains.

Treatment engagement evaluates participation quality while identifying factors that support or hinder involvement in therapeutic activities and recovery processes.

Recommendations outline ongoing treatment needs while providing guidance for continuing care and service coordination that supports sustained recovery and growth.

Insurance Documentation Guides

Specialized documentation templates meet insurance requirements while ensuring appropriate reimbursement for group therapy services and supporting access to care for group members.

Medical necessity justification demonstrates need for group therapy while providing clinical rationale that supports insurance coverage and authorization for treatment services.

Treatment goal documentation specifies measurable objectives while ensuring that group therapy targets align with insurance-covered conditions and approved treatment modalities.

Progress reporting provides required updates while documenting therapeutic benefit and continued need for services that support ongoing authorization and payment.

Outcome measurement uses standardized instruments while providing objective data that demonstrates treatment effectiveness and medical necessity for insurance review purposes.

Service coordination documents integration with other treatments while showing how group therapy complements individual interventions and supports overall care planning.

Case Example: Insurance Documentation Strategy

Our anxiety disorders program developed systematic insurance documentation that supported coverage while demonstrating group therapy medical necessity and treatment effectiveness.

Initial authorization requests included detailed clinical assessments documenting anxiety severity, functional impairment, and specific deficits that group therapy would address through peer support and skill development.

Progress reports provided quarterly updates using GAD-7 scores and functional assessment data while demonstrating measurable improvement and continued medical necessity for ongoing group participation.

Treatment planning documentation showed how group therapy goals aligned with individual treatment objectives while providing evidence of coordinated care and appropriate service utilization.

Outcome reporting used standardized measures to demonstrate anxiety reduction and improved functioning while providing objective evidence of treatment effectiveness for insurance review.

Appeals support maintained detailed records of clinical decision-making while providing documentation necessary for challenging coverage denials or authorization limitations.

This systematic approach resulted in 95% authorization success rates while ensuring appropriate reimbursement for group therapy services.

Electronic Documentation Systems

Modern healthcare environments increasingly rely on electronic health records that require adaptation of documentation templates while maintaining clinical quality and regulatory compliance.

Template integration adapts group therapy documentation for electronic systems while ensuring that standardized formats translate effectively to digital platforms and maintain clinical utility.

Workflow optimization streamlines documentation processes while reducing administrative burden and improving efficiency without compromising clinical quality or regulatory compliance.

Data sharing enables communication between providers while protecting confidentiality and ensuring that group therapy information contributes appropriately to coordinated care planning.

Quality assurance monitors documentation completeness while identifying areas for improvement and ensuring that electronic records meet both clinical and regulatory standards.

Backup procedures protect against data loss while ensuring continuity of care and maintaining access to essential clinical information during system failures or transitions.

Legal and Ethical Considerations

Group therapy documentation involves complex legal and ethical issues that require careful attention while balancing transparency with confidentiality and protection of both individual and group privacy.

Confidentiality protection ensures appropriate privacy while allowing necessary information sharing that supports treatment coordination and emergency care when needed.

Informed consent addresses documentation practices while ensuring that group members understand how their information will be recorded and shared with appropriate parties.

Regulatory compliance meets federal and state requirements while ensuring that documentation practices support rather than hinder appropriate clinical care and treatment planning.

Professional standards maintain ethical documentation while supporting best practices and evidence-based care that protects both patients and providers from liability.

Quality improvement uses documentation data appropriately while protecting privacy and ensuring that information supports program development rather than individual identification.

Documentation Training and Support

Effective documentation requires ongoing education while building organizational capacity for quality record-keeping that supports both clinical care and regulatory compliance.

Initial training provides foundation skills while ensuring that all staff understand documentation requirements and standards for group therapy practice and record-keeping.

Ongoing education maintains current knowledge while addressing changes in regulations, standards, and best practices that affect documentation requirements and procedures.

Quality monitoring evaluates documentation quality while providing feedback and support for improvement in record-keeping practices and clinical communication.

Supervision support provides guidance for complex situations while ensuring that documentation decisions reflect appropriate clinical judgment and professional standards.

System improvement refines documentation processes while building efficiency and effectiveness that supports clinical care rather than creating administrative burden.

Moving Forward with Documentation

Effective documentation represents the bridge between excellent clinical care and professional accountability that supports both individual treatment and advancement of group therapy as evidence-based practice. Your commitment to quality record-keeping demonstrates your professionalism while protecting the individuals you serve.

The templates and systems you develop become resources for other professionals while contributing to the standardization and improvement of group therapy documentation across healthcare settings and professional communities.

Documentation Essentials

- SOAP and DAP progress note formats provide structured templates while ensuring consistent documentation that meets clinical and regulatory requirements
- Attendance tracking and behavioral observation forms capture participation patterns while providing data for treatment planning and outcome evaluation
- Incident report templates ensure appropriate crisis documentation while supporting quality improvement and legal protection for all parties
- Outcome summary reports synthesize progress data while providing evidence for treatment effectiveness and continued care authorization
- Insurance documentation guides support appropriate reimbursement while demonstrating medical necessity and treatment coordination
- Electronic systems integration and legal considerations ensure modern documentation while maintaining confidentiality and regulatory compliance

Reference

1. Burlingame, G. M., McClendon, D. T., & Yang, C. (2018). Cohesion in group therapy: A meta-analysis. *Psychotherapy*, 55(4), 384-398.
2. Peplau, H. E. (1991). *Interpersonal relations in nursing: A conceptual frame of reference for psychodynamic nursing.* Springer Publishing Company.
3. Orlando, I. J. (1972). *The discipline and teaching of nursing process: An evaluative study.* G. P. Putnam's Sons.
4. Watson, J. (2008). *Nursing: The philosophy and science of caring* (Rev. ed.). University Press of Colorado.
5. Travelbee, J. (1971). *Interpersonal aspects of nursing* (2nd ed.). F. A. Davis Company.
6. Yalom, I. D., & Leszcz, M. (2020). *The theory and practice of group psychotherapy* (6th ed.). Basic Books.
7. Tuckman, B. W., & Jensen, M. A. C. (1977). Stages of small-group development revisited. *Group & Organization Studies*, 2(4), 419-427.
8. MacKenzie, K. R. (1983). The clinical application of a group climate measure. In R. R. Dies & K. R. MacKenzie (Eds.), *Advances in group psychotherapy: Integrating research and practice* (pp. 159-170). International Universities Press.
9. Lese, K. P., & MacNair-Semands, R. R. (2000). The Therapeutic Factors Inventory: Development of a scale. *Group*, 24(4), 303-317.
10. Beck, A. T., Rush, A. J., Shaw, B. F., & Emery, G. (1979). *Cognitive therapy of depression.* Guilford Press.
11. Dobson, K. S., & Dozois, D. J. A. (2019). *Handbook of cognitive-behavioral therapies* (4th ed.). Guilford Press.
12. Wright, J. H., Brown, G. K., Thase, M. E., & Basco, M. R. (2017). *Learning cognitive-behavior therapy: An illustrated guide* (2nd ed.). American Psychiatric Publishing.
13. Linehan, M. M. (2014). *DBT skills training manual* (2nd ed.). Guilford Press.
14. Siegel, R. D., Germer, C. K., & Olendzki, A. (2009). Mindfulness: What is it? Where did it come from? In F. Didonna (Ed.), *Clinical handbook of mindfulness* (pp. 17-35). Springer.
15. Linehan, M. M. (2014). *DBT skills training handouts and worksheets* (2nd ed.). Guilford Press.
16. Gratz, K. L., & Tull, M. T. (2011). Emotion regulation as a mechanism of change in acceptance- and mindfulness-based treatments. In R. A. Baer (Ed.), *Assessing mindfulness and acceptance processes in clients* (pp. 107-133). Context Press.
17. Koerner, K. (2012). *Doing dialectical behavior therapy: A practical guide.* Guilford Press.

18. Goyal, M., Singh, S., Sibinga, E. M., Gould, N. F., Rowland-Seymour, A., Sharma, R., Berger, Z., Sleicher, D., Maron, D. D., Shihab, H. M., Ranasinghe, P. D., Linn, S., Saha, S., Bass, E. B., & Haythornthwaite, J. A. (2014). Meditation programs for psychological stress and well-being: A systematic review and meta-analysis. *JAMA Internal Medicine*, 174(3), 357-368.
19. Patel, M. X., Doku, V., & Tennakoon, L. (2003). Challenges in recruitment of research participants. *Advances in Psychiatric Treatment*, 9(3), 229-238.
20. Semahegn, A., Torpey, K., Manu, A., Assefa, N., Tesfaye, G., & Ankomah, A. (2020). Psychotropic medication non-adherence and its associated factors among patients with major psychiatric disorders: A systematic review and meta-analysis. *Systematic Reviews*, 9(1), 17.
21. Velligan, D. I., Weiden, P. J., Sajatovic, M., Scott, J., Carpenter, D., Ross, R., Docherty, J. P., & Expert Consensus Panel on Adherence Problems in Serious and Persistent Mental Illness. (2009). The expert consensus guideline series: Adherence problems in patients with serious and persistent mental illness. *Journal of Clinical Psychiatry*, 70(4), 1-46.
22. Garrick, J., & Garrick, F. (2001). An integrated model for adolescent inpatient group therapy. *Journal of Psychiatric and Mental Health Nursing*, 8(6), 487-494.
23. Blake, H., Mo, P., Malik, S., & Thomas, S. (2009). How effective are physical activity interventions for alleviating depressive symptoms in older people? A systematic review. *Clinical Rehabilitation*, 23(10), 873-887.
24. Woods, B., O'Philbin, L., Farrell, E. M., Spector, A. E., & Orrell, M. (2018). Reminiscence therapy for dementia. *Cochrane Database of Systematic Reviews*, 3(3), CD001120.
25. Spector, A., Thorgrimsen, L., Woods, B., Royan, L., Davies, S., Butterworth, M., & Orrell, M. (2003). Efficacy of an evidence-based cognitive stimulation therapy programme for people with dementia: Randomised controlled trial. *British Journal of Psychiatry*, 183(3), 248-254.
26. Drake, R. E., Mueser, K. T., Brunette, M. F., & McHugo, G. J. (2004). A review of treatments for people with severe mental illnesses and co-occurring substance use disorders. *Psychiatric Rehabilitation Journal*, 27(4), 360-374.
27. Sue, D. W., & Sue, D. (2019). *Counseling the culturally diverse: Theory and practice* (8th ed.). John Wiley & Sons.
28. Forsyth, D. R. (2018). *Group dynamics* (7th ed.). Cengage Learning.
29. Kaplan, S. G., & Wheeler, E. G. (2011). Medical emergency procedures for the group psychotherapy setting. *International Journal of Group Psychotherapy*, 61(3), 367-387.
30. Yalom, I. D., & Leszcz, M. (2020). Process and outcome in group therapy. In *The theory and practice of group psychotherapy* (6th ed., pp. 71-115). Basic Books.

31. American Psychiatric Association. (2022). *Diagnostic and statistical manual of mental disorders* (5th ed., text rev.). American Psychiatric Publishing.
32. Stuart, G. W. (2018). *Principles and practice of psychiatric nursing* (11th ed.). Elsevier.

33. Beck, A. T., Steer, R. A., & Brown, G. K. (1996). *Manual for the Beck Depression Inventory-II*. Psychological Corporation.
34. Kroenke, K., Spitzer, R. L., & Williams, J. B. (2001). The PHQ-9: Validity of a brief depression severity measure. *Journal of General Internal Medicine*, 16(9), 606-613.
35. Wing, J. K., Beevor, A. S., Curtis, R. H., Park, S. B., Hadden, S., & Burns, A. (1998). Health of the Nation Outcome Scales (HoNOS): Research and development. *British Journal of Psychiatry*, 172(1), 11-18.

www.ingramcontent.com/pod-product-compliance
Lightning Source LLC
Chambersburg PA
CBHW080429230426
43662CB00015B/2223